NEWTON FREE LIBRARY
330 HOMER ST.
NEWTON, MA 024 P9-CFP-091

WITHDRAWN

NEWTON FREE LIBRARY
HOMER ST

SQUARE ONE

SQUARE ONE

RETURNING TO LIFE AND COMPETITIVE RUNNING AFTER MY DEVASTATING STROKE

DIRK VLIEKS

FOREWORD BY AMBY BURFOOT

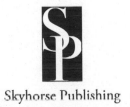

Skyhorse Publishing

Copyright © 2017 by Dirk Vlieks

All rights reserved. No part of this book may be reproduced in any manner without the express written consent of the publisher, except in the case of brief excerpts in critical reviews or articles. All inquiries should be addressed to Skyhorse Publishing, 307 West 36th Street, 11th Floor, New York, NY 10018.

Skyhorse Publishing books may be purchased in bulk at special discounts for sales promotion, corporate gifts, fund-raising, or educational purposes. Special editions can also be created to specifications. For details, contact the Special Sales Department, Skyhorse Publishing, 307 West 36th Street, 11th Floor, New York, NY 10018 or info@skyhorsepublishing.com.

Skyhorse® and Skyhorse Publishing® are registered trademarks of Skyhorse Publishing, Inc.®, a Delaware corporation.

Visit our website at www.skyhorsepublishing.com.

10 9 8 7 6 5 4 3 2 1

Library of Congress Cataloging-in-Publication Data is available on file.

Cover design by Tom Lau
Front cover photos by Kelsey Vlieks (left) and Ute Vlieks (center, right)
Back cover photo by Ute Vlieks

Print ISBN: 978-1-5107-2100-5
Ebook ISBN: 978-1-5107-2101-2

Printed in the United States of America

Dedication

To Kelsey and the girls, Ellie and Anna

TABLE OF CONTENTS

Foreword

I met Dirk Vlieks while doing something we both have spent a fair amount of time doing—running. When I first spotted him walking herky-jerky across the parking lot at Haley Farm State Park in Groton, Connecticut, I wondered who he was and what was wrong with him.

On this late September morning, perfect for running, I had gathered with a handful of serious runner-friends at Haley Farm, a gorgeous park with long, winding trails and views of nearby Long Island Sound. It was the perfect place for a Sunday morning run.

Dirk didn't look like he would fit in with our group. I thought that he might be just ambling along on a solo walk. It didn't take Dirk long to disabuse me of my mistaken notion. He took off on a seven-mile run with the rest of us and more than held his own. In fact, once he broke into his running stride, I couldn't help but marvel at how smoothly he moved along.

Certainly, his strong stride belied what he had been through and how much he had accomplished to get back to running.

After that first run, I got to know Dirk a bit better and slowly learned his story. Not that Dirk told me much at first about his life-threatening, on-the-run episode, or how much he had struggled to return to his running ways.

Dirk's not the kind of guy who spends a lot of time looking back or talking about himself. I admire that. Still, I did learn that he was new to the Mystic, Connecticut, running scene, and quite serious about his training and racing.

I gradually pieced together that Dirk had been a serious triathlon competitor with a number of Ironman finishes. The day I first saw him at Haley Farm, it was easy to see that he had been through something. I was curious to uncover more.

On subsequent runs, I noticed that his gait wasn't the only strange thing about him. When he spoke, I missed some of his words. They came out a bit garbled and difficult to understand. Still, his story came through.

I learned more on each of our runs and at several races. It was clear that Dirk loved to run. He popped up here, there, and everywhere local runners gathered.

One day he told me he was writing a book. That particularly piqued my curiosity, since I am also a writer. Yet the more I heard from Dirk, the more I realized that there were big gaps in my understanding of his background and medical history.

Another time we met for lunch at the Mystic Market to talk more about books and running. Dirk told me he had completed a rough draft of his book and asked me if I would be willing to read it. Of course I agreed to. Now at last I could learn all the details I hadn't pieced together yet.

Reading *Square One* certainly filled in the holes. It's an unblinking account of what happened to Dirk in the middle of the Honu Half Ironman. One minute he was jostling for position on the bike ride, the next he was collapsing to the ground after a tumor burst and caused a massive stroke.

His courageous story will no doubt impress every reader, and not just because Dirk was talented and disciplined enough to make it to Honu. No, this is one of those unbelievable comeback stories. Dirk was down—way down—but he refused to stay there. In the often difficult days and years since Honu, he has worked his way back to a very close approximation of his former self.

And not only that, he and his wife have had two beautiful girls (twins), and he has maintained his commitment to health and fitness. In fact, he's back to running marathons again. You can't go much farther than that.

Amby Burfoot
Runner's World Editor At Large
1968 Boston Marathon winner
Mystic, Connecticut

Introduction

I loved triathlon because I loved pushing boundaries. I felt there was no better way to test myself. Once I had my first taste, I knew immediately that triathlon was the ideal complement to what drove me—the perfect sport with the perfect blend of exertion and adrenaline and discipline. I thought it was the ultimate challenge, the most demanding thing I would ever face.

I was wrong.

In a lifetime of looking for challenges, I learned quickly there were a few I'd have preferred not to face. Learning to walk again at age thirty-four was harder. So was learning to eat and speak again. Those were just a bit more challenging than anything thrown at me by an Ironman.

But maybe everything I had done before "the event"—the midrace stroke in 2006 that sent me to edge of the precipice, where my life hung tenuously by the thinnest of threads—had prepared me for what lay ahead. That day in Hawaii I was transformed in a few brief moments from athlete to helpless infant, from the lead group of cyclists to an intensive care unit where doctors felt certain I would not make it, from trying to qualify for the big race to simply staying alive.

Maybe triathlon saved me.

If you've never thought of attempting to swim, then bike, then run without interruption over any distance, your first question is obvious.

"Why?"

If you ramp up the distances, Ironman distances, between seventy and one hundred forty miles for a day's outing, your next question will be, "Are you out of your mind?"

For me, my first triathlon was an irresistible Siren Song. Once I heard it, I couldn't get it out of my mind. And nothing in my life was ever the same again.

I love triathlon. I'm not trying to be disingenuous when I talk about how difficult it is to finish one while I call attention to the fact that I've finished many. I don't believe in ostentation or showing off. These races are difficult for everyone, plain and simple. In many ways, they are ordeals to be finished, not events to be savored. But in other ways, they are celebrations of your physical strength and mental tenacity. That's the point, and that's why tens of thousands of athletes, men and women of all ages, take them on every year.

Finish an iron-distance triathlon and you are on top of the world, exhausted, elated, and ready for anything that life will throw at you in the real world. An oft-quoted saying among competitors is "triathlon doesn't build character, it reveals it."

Read what a few others have said about triathlons and you'll get the idea.

Mark Allen, a six-time Ironman world champion, said this about the Ironman, the competition that started this whole thing: "Until you face your fears you don't move to the other side, where you find the power."

John Collins, known as the "Father of Ironman," put it this way: "The pain is temporary, the memories will last the rest of your life."

Add what two-time Ironman world champion Chris McCormack said about it: "You don't play triathlon. You play soccer; it's fun. You play baseball. Triathlon is work that can leave you crumpled in a heap, puking by the roadside. It's the physical brutality of climbing Mount Everest without the great view from the top of the world. What kind of person keeps coming back for more of that?"

I kept coming back.

I loved it and still do. There's the elation at the finish, of course, but there is also the growing confidence as you train, the self-assurance that comes with the discipline you need, the friends you train with, the common bonds, pushing your limits, knowing yourself. The list is long.

The idea for Ironman started in 1977 with a friendly argument in Hawaii between swimmers and runners over who was fitter, a pretty standard dispute that's been around probably for as long as people have been swimming and running. That's when John Collins, a US Navy commander, upped the stakes, pointing out that *Sports Illustrated* had asserted that Belgian cyclist Eddy Merckx was perhaps the fittest athlete around.

Collins tossed in that maybe cyclists are fitter than either swimmers or runners.

And so the seed was planted, and it quickly grew into what would be called the Ironman: a 2.4-mile ocean swim followed by a 112-mile bike ride topped off by a marathon, 26.2 miles of final torture.

Fifteen men started the first Ironman on February 18, 1978. Twelve finished, and nothing has been the same since.

A *Sports Illustrated* article following the 1979 race started the buzz building, but probably nothing did more to burn the image of what the race can do to competitors—and to raise interest in it worldwide—than Julie Moss's 1982 finish, where a national audience watching ABC's *Wide World of Sports* saw her collapse so torturously close to the finish and struggle to hold her lead. Less than ten yards from the line, she collapsed for the final time. As Moss lay writhing in the darkness, she was passed by Kathleen McCartney, who was unaware she had won the race.

Moss became the poster child for the Ironman, an indelible symbol of everything it took. Her finish did more to put Ironman on the map than anything else.

I was ten years old when Julie Moss brought Ironman into the public consciousness. It would take me a while get to the finish line in Hawaii, but I eventually would.

I've always enjoyed moving and competing, and in my peripatetic early childhood, with family hopping from Ohio to Canada and around Europe every two or three years, sports gave me a way to focus. At first, in Europe, it was skiing, but when we moved back to the states when I was ten, skiing took a backseat to tennis, which consumed me all through high school and onto college, where I played Division I at St. Mary's College in Moraga, California.

A challenge from my older brother, Olaf, had sent me to the courts, motivated me. He was a good player, and he turned to me the summer before I hit sixth grade and said I'd never make the high school varsity team as a freshman. That was the only fuel I needed. I made the varsity as a freshman and didn't look back.

I loved everything about tennis.

I even took it a step further after college and began playing professionally in some international tournaments. But the slashing back-and-forth of years of tennis took its toll on my knees fairly early. A year after I graduated from St. Mary's in 1996, after playing in a tournament in Brazil, my knees were shot, and I came back home for some rehab work.

"Find something to do where you go straight," a physical therapist told me.

And so the story begins. Enter triathlon. I had found another passion.

I have never thought of myself as an elite athlete. I was simply wired to compete, able to relish the long hours of training, to actually look forward to them. It takes a lot of hours to get to the finish line of an Ironman. I spent quite a few of those hours with guys who were Olympic and world-class competitors, and their fervor for the sport wore off on me. I saw what it took.

Basically, a triathlon goes something like this, no matter what the distance:

You enter the swim leg, always the first segment, in a pack. No matter how much you try to avoid it, you'll be kicked or elbowed, unintentionally for the most part. There is always a lot of adrenaline pumping. But soon people pick their lines and the pack spreads out. You begin swimming, find your rhythm, mindful of breathing and stroke and cadence, conscious that you will be pushing yourself for the rest of the day but staying below the line where you will burn out too early. It's a long race and a delicate balance.

Next, you emerge from the water and head for your bike, the transition zone for changing usually mildly chaotic and sometimes jarring. But you must simply focus, find your bike, get your shoes and helmet, and head out. The pack has spread even more by then, so the beginning of the bike leg is not nearly as raucous as the start of the swim. You ride, concentrate, and again find the rhythm. Too much and you don't finish. Not enough and you finish poorly.

The final leg is always the run. Pushing pedals in a set cadence wears on legs in a much different way than running does. If you've trained properly, the transition from pedaling to striding is relatively easy. If you haven't, the moment your feet hit the road for the run, your legs buckle and turn to goo. Your quads burn and refuse to engage. You stumble. If you have done the proper training, your stride will come quickly and you'll head for the finish.

Sounds relatively simple, but of course it's not.

These races don't take place in air-conditioned arenas. They are outside, and that might mean ocean waves and whitecaps, tides going against you, humidity, high winds in your face, hills. It might mean being cut off by an oblivious biker or being kicked in the face by the guy in front of you on the swim.

Each leg has its own peculiarities. The swim offers the jostling. The bike leg, the challenge of trying to ingest enough nutrients to keep on the right side of the envelope, to fuel yourself to make it to the finish. And then there are the unexpected issues like having your goggles kicked off and flat tires and crashes. Running will bring joint and muscles issues and blisters.

If I had a favorite leg, I guess it would be the run (fewer complications).

I never set precise goals for myself, but I always shot for a top finish. You just never know how you will feel in any particular race and the mechanical wild cards are simply too hard to predict. But I did go into each race with confidence.

Confidence comes from training, sometimes up to sixteen hours a week, and knowing you're ready. Eight-hour bike rides, two-hour swims, hours of running. The discipline was part of my life. And it was part of the lives of the people I trained with who were as crazy about it as I was. That always helps.

After my stroke, when the biggest challenge of my life had begun, all this effort would come home to roost and help immeasurably. And so would the many friends I met and raced against.

When I was in my lowest hours after my stroke, fighting the darkness that would sometimes threaten my resolve, I'd draw on how I felt as I approached an Ironman finish, twenty-four miles into the run. In front of me would always be someone I'd been trying to catch for the last hour, one more person to pass. Maybe we'd been dueling all day.

That was when I would tell myself one more time, "Kick it in and pass that guy."

Usually I would. My stroke, my ultimate challenge, would be yet another chance to kick it in.

In a way, that helped.

One

THE EVENT

Rituals are always comforting, and mine always worked.

I had a subtle and practiced ritual before each race that I rarely changed. I would begin to settle into myself the night before, slowly making the transition from genial to focused. By the time I went to bed, I'd be at the point where I spoke only when I needed to. Before I drifted calmly off to sleep, I would put on my game face and go through the race mentally, imagining how I'd feel at certain points. Before bed, I'd lay out everything I needed the next day on the floor so I'd see it and count it when I woke up —the swim goggles, the nutrition packets and water bottles, the things that would sustain me the next day.

The night before the Honu Half-Ironman triathlon in Kailua-Kona, Hawaii, in June of 2006, I dropped off to sleep satisfied I was ready for what would be a qualifier for the actual Ironman, the big race I loved. I had finished the full Ford World Championship Ironman at Kona the year before and was trying to requalify.

On race day morning, I had concentrated on the phases ahead and the hours I'd be working, controlling my adrenaline surges as much as I could to preserve energy.

There were patterns in every race I knew that would insert themselves during the long day ahead, some highs—an unexpected surge of energy on the bike, for example. And there would be brief moments of despair—being passed on the run when I hadn't expected it. For the most part, I'd simply fold into the race, lost in concentration. The emotional cycle was familiar to me and, in a way, comforting: the adrenaline, the tight nerves, the focus, the surges.

Then there was the finish. Since I never set out to win a race, only to do my best, I never had the crashing emotions some top finishers experience. Since I trained to do my best and was comfortable with the challenges, the finish was nearly always a time of great relief and happiness.

The end of a race did not fail to bring what I can only describe as a wonderful and serene wave of euphoria—an almost overwhelming sense that I had again pushed myself and had accomplished what I set out to do. That's the reason I race.

I always loved that euphoria of the finish. I ate it up it and looked forward to it. I would let go for a bit and let the feeling of accomplishment wash over me, I'd indulge myself in pride of accomplishment. Postrace was always a great time. Usually my wife, Kelsey, and I would have a slow and relaxed dinner with friends, all of us laughing and feeling the same. It's incomparable, that feeling. It's wonderful.

I never got to the euphoria phase on June 3, 2006. I never had the delicious dinner or hugged my wife or joked with friends. Around the time I should have been digging into a delicious dinner and relishing the day's events, I was simply trying to stay alive.

When I stood on the beach in Kona that day, I had gone through my prerace ritual as I always did more than fifty times. I was in full game-face mode. I was ready. My legs felt great and I was motivated.

My goal for the race was to simply not hold back on anything and to go as hard as I could, when I could. I wanted to race smart, that is, to maintain the rhythm and balance of energy over the hours I'd be pushing and not burn out too early. The funny thing is, when "the event" took me down, I had not yet really pushed myself.

I always sleep well before races, and that day was no exception. And keeping with that, I got up early to enjoy a strong cup of coffee and mentally go through the race.

By that point I was happy with my training. Working up to each race, I always looked for ways to improve, a more efficient swim stroke, better bike cadence, smarter run strategy—there was always something I could improve. Luckily, I always had great training partners, people who wouldn't look at you open-mouthed when you said you wanted to do an extra mile of swimming or another hour of running. They were great company, and we enjoyed pushing one another, yet another side benefit of triathlon.

These partners would prove invaluable later.

I'd left SFO from United Airlines Gate 80 for a direct flight to Kona, the Big Island, with little fanfare, just a few "good lucks" and "do wells" from coworkers, clients, and friends. They were used to the scene, and I never liked to make a big deal out of a race anyway. When I got to Kona, I began to settle into the prerace ritual with a few short bike rides to get my legs moving and a few sprints to get the heart pumping a bit, but nothing too long. Before the race it was always "legs up," nothing more than a short swim.

There were always familiar faces at a race, regulars who love the competition and eat it up. Before the race there's not a lot of socializing other than a quick cup of coffee and chat. Everyone has the game-face look.

I prepared as I always had, and I felt great and ready and excited—as I always had. There were no ominous signs auguring what would happen in a matter of hours down the highway as I stood at the starting line on the beach wearing bib number 789 with more than a thousand other competitors.

The weather that morning was cool, which is always preferable. The wind was light and the water fairly quiet. I heard the wind picked up later, but by then I was out of the race.

As the swim got off to its usually chaotic start, I picked my line and tried to follow it. With so many other swimmers trying to do the same thing, there was the inevitable jostling. The trick is to stay cool and centered. The mildly controlled chaos is inevitable when there were so many amped-up athletes about to unleash combined tens of thousands of hours of training. On the beach, most of us would by that time be making idle silly chit-chat, just to keep our minds off what lay ahead.

Among the supporters at the start were, of course, my wonderful wife, Kelsey, herself an endurance athlete, and her friend Dixie Hauth, who was on hand to encourage her husband, Chris Hauth, a former Olympic swimmer and my training partner and good friend. Kelsey and Dixie planned to follow us through various phases and yell an occasional blast of inspiration if they saw me or Chris during the race, which as a half-Ironman would comprise a 1.2-mile swim, 56-mile bike, and 13.5-mile run.

As the gun sounded on the beach, we were off, a thousand highly trained triathletes with one goal in mind, finish and finish well. I did what I always did, blasting out quickly to get ahead of the clamoring masses. Three minutes into the swim, I felt fine. I was out of the water in 30.31, a good time. A friend later gave me a great photo of me as I emerged from the swim leg. I definitely had my game face on, my eyes locked ahead, but my stride was open and I was in attack mode for sure. I was happy to be out and heading for my bike without any issues.

I was ready for the bike leg, something I had worked on with a laser focus leading up to the race. This was where I planned to put the hammer down and insert myself among the leaders. Chris and I would sometimes do 100-mile training rides through the Northern California hills to get ready for Hawaii.

The transition zone, where athletes scramble to their bikes and try to get off as smoothly as possible, was fairly clutter-free. I knew where my bike, an Interloc Slipstream SC, was and headed right to it. I wanted to get out as fast as I could. I felt like the bike phase was where I would lock in on focus and give everything I had.

I had planned everything down to the final detail, bringing with me GU and GU20 for nutrition and other necessities like bananas and salt pills and, of course, plenty of water. The whole idea was to make sure the vital sugars I needed to take in worked well together. Stomach cramps and worse are a midrace nightmare. Having a massive stroke midrace can be a bit of a bummer, as well, I would learn later.

As I headed into the ride, my rhythm and pace building just as I had planned, the chills from the morning swim were replaced by increasingly warmer air. The wind was from the side, certainly better than a long slog into a strong headwind.

About fifty minutes and about eighteen miles in and working smoothly up Queen K (Kaahumanu) Highway, I began to feel something was amiss. I was just a bit off. It was an odd feeling, certainly, when I had trained so well and planned so meticulously. It wasn't as if I were jolted with a sudden pain. I began to feel dizzy, which in itself is fairly common with water in your inner ear from the swim trying to free itself as you move your head from side to side. That had happened before, and it had always gone away after a few miles on the bike.

This time it didn't.

It latched on and settled in, which was quite a different feeling from past rides. My vision began to blur. It got worse with each push of the pedal. For the first time ever, in more than dozens of triathlons, the thought that I needed to stop crept in. By that point I was approaching the lead pack, which was just heading into a downhill turn.

As I watched the lead pack I had so much wanted to catch heading into the turn, I gave up, conceding the race and knowing only that it would be safer to get off my bike near people rather than out somewhere in no-man's-land where nobody would see me in trouble.

I felt like shit, and I started looking for a place to pull off the course. Queen's Highway was lined on both sides with black lava fields, not a great place to lie down. I saw a patch of grass near the Hawi town line that looked like a good place to stop. I had never dropped out of a race before. Stopping to rest had never been in any playbook I had followed. I knew that once I got off the bike, it was over for me. This wasn't a time where I could get off, rest, regroup, and head back into the fray. It was over. And at that point I didn't care. Something was seriously awry and I could sense it. I was thirty-three years old and in the best shape of my life. I thought I was dying.

My first thought was of Kelsey. I didn't know what was going on, but I knew it was serious. What ultimately happened was the furthest thing from my mind as I pulled off the road, but I knew I was in crisis.

I saw the grass patch and pulled off, unsnapping my helmet, and using my bike to steady myself as I lay down because I had begun to stagger by that time.

That was when the first of several very fortunate blessings occurred. As I was reeling, race director Jimmy Riccitello passed by on the back of a Harley, scanning racers for problems and making sure things were running smoothly, as race directors must do.

"I need some help," I yelled out as I struggled to keep calm. Things were getting worse very quickly. My uneasy dismount and my plea for help to Jimmy were enough to have him tell the Harley driver to pull over, but he was not initially alarmed.

Jimmy, who became a great friend, would later tell me that he didn't realize I was in trouble, at least physically.

"You looked normal," he said. Of course I was anything but.

As I lay on that patch of grass I told him, as my words by then were beginning to slur, that my head hurt. I told him I thought I was dying.

I told him to call Kelsey and tell her I loved her.

Riccitello called into Race Operations on his handheld radio and told them he needed help immediately but got no response from that remote spot. He tried his cell phone, and again, nothing.

His driver tried as well and was able to get through. Help was on the way, she was told. Race Operations had heard Riccitello's first radio message.

As I was lying on the ground, Riccitello checked my heart rate monitor. It read 60. At that point in the race, after the swim and almost twenty miles into a strenuous bike ride, it should have been around 140 or 150.

That was the first time the alarm rang loudly, the first time the fateful word would be mentioned.

"I need someone out here fast," Riccitello said on a second, more urgent call. "We might have a stroke victim here."

My head still hurt and my vision was fading quickly. I asked Jimmy three more times to make sure he called Kelsey, to make sure he told her I loved her.

I could hear Riccitello asking racers passing by if they were doctors. That was one of the last clear memories I have of that day. Everything after that for a very long time would be a fast-moving blur—a mix of brief moments of clarity and nightmarish darkness.

Finally, Riccitello saw someone he knew, and she pulled over, which was a blessing. By stopping midrace, she had done something many others would have found unimaginable. Imagine training hundreds of hours for a race and stopping to help. That simple act was a tremendous sacrifice—and wonderfully unselfish.

She was one of several blessings that day. I could have had the stroke during the swim and not been seen in the frenzy. I could have had it on a forty-mile-an-hour downhill section with lava fields on both sides earlier on the bike leg. Other injections of good karma would arrive in due time.

My Good Samaritan made sure I was lying on my back as medical help from Race Operations arrived. I was put on a stretcher and slipped gently into the back of a van. Medics started an IV, and the van turned across Queen K Highway and headed back to the medical tent at race headquarters.

I was drifting in and out of consciousness.

By then, ahead of where I was now lying on the road getting medical attention, Kelsey and Dixie had been among the cheerful crowd standing under the palm trees in front of the Mauna Kea Hotel down from Hapuna Beach, waiting for the cyclists to pass. They saw Chris in the lead group of four and thought I would not be far behind.

I have often thought that watching a long triathlon, trying to keep up with me, was harder than actually racing it. But Kelsey always did it and always seemed to manage to grab a spot where she could yell some encouragement. She was there that day when I got out of the water, standing in the transition zone and yelling, "Pick it up, honey."

They didn't spot me as Chris and the lead group swept past, but they weren't worried. Any number of things could have been the reason. A flat tire, a mechanical problem, a crash maybe, and with more than a thousand racers, they might simply have missed me in the packs of cyclists flashing by. Of course, the thought of a major medical crisis was not among the reasons.

Kelsey called her mother in Connecticut and asked her to use an online tracking system on the Ironman website to find out where I was. Her mom called back a minute later and said she could not find me. That was the first small injection of anxiety on what would be a terrifying day for Kelsey and our families.

Kelsey and Dixie decided to head for race headquarters to see what was going on. They parked their rental car and were headed to the Fairmont Hotel when they passed the medical tent. That's when blessing number three of the day dropped in. Kelsey glanced into the tent through an open flap and noticed a pair of shaven legs flopped on a cot—my legs. She recognized them instantly.

By that time, I was unconscious.

Kelsey, a physical therapist who had completed graduate school a year earlier and was working at a rehabilitation outpatient facility near our home in California, knew all too intimately the signs. Despite the tremendous shock, Kelsey snapped quickly into an unemotional and professional mode. Dixie began crying.

"I knew instantly what had happened when I saw your left side was paralyzed. That's when I said my first prayer," Kelsey told me later.

It was strangely quiet in the tent, usually the scene of an athlete being treated for dehydration or road rash or the unusual medically inconsequential irritations of a long race with many participants. Certainly not strokes among this group of hyperfit athletes.

A nurse noticed Kelsey and asked if she was my wife. No one else was speaking, certainly not me.

It was not good.

Following established protocol, the emergency doctors on hand began what would be an IV drip of two liters of a dextrose and saline solution and pricked me to test my response to pain stimuli. I was unresponsive. They found that I would move my right hand and foot when asked, but nothing on my left side.

On hand was Franklin Marcus, a cardiac anesthesiologist, who was medical director of the race that day. Used to treating something like forty racers during a race like the Kona, he'd never seen anything as severe as my case in the twenty-five years he'd been a volunteer. Usually he treated racers for dehydration and electrolyte issues brought on by cyclists being unable to drink as much as they should have because high winds required they grip the handles tightly.

He pulled Kelsey away from my side at the cot and outside the tent.

"This is bad," he told her. "There seems to be a large amount of internal bleeding."

Then came blessing number four. Assisting for the first time was a recently graduated neurologist—uncommon in a group of volunteers usually comprised of family practitioners and sports medicine guys. He was so fresh from medical school that he had not yet seen an acute stroke, but he noticed that my symptoms were textbook classic.

I began to slip into total unconsciousness, which an on-edge Dr. Marcus noticed immediately. Kelsey stood behind him yelling at me to stay awake.

Dr. Marcus immediately ordered the medical van to take me to the emergency room at the small forty-bed North Hawaii Community Hospital in nearby Waimea for more tests.

I was put on life support as soon as I was quickly but gingerly brought into the ER.

I had suffered a massive hemorrhagic stroke, a nearly always fatal eruption. At that early point no one was sure precisely where it had occurred, but somewhere in my brain a weakened blood vessel had ruptured. A torrent of blood was literally flooding my brain cavity near the critical area that controlled my breathing.

Survivors of these massive strokes usually end up in a permanent coma.

I was intubated, a long flexible tube inserted in my throat to allow a machine to do my breathing for me.

Much later, I would remember dreams of being trapped underwater, desperate for breath. In the dream I'd occasionally break through to the surface and gasp for breath. Then I would sink once more into the darkness.

It was odd, that small spark of memory of nearly suffocating. For years I would not be able to dream about anything, and I would fervently wish each night for some relief from troubled sleep.

The severity of a day that had begun as so many other race days with hope and excitement was settling in. Kelsey, still in professional mode, did not cry but was slowly being overcome with nausea. Dixie had left to find Chris at the finish, and when they rejoined Kelsey, they found her shivering at my bedside from shock and the chill of the air conditioning.

The ER physician returned with the CT scan results. I had had a brainstem hemorrhage with an intraventricular extension. The rupture had occurred in an area of the brain where all cognitive motor functions are controlled, things like vision, certain sensations, and the ability to walk and talk. It was as if a perfect storm dropped into Times Square on New Year's Eve.

A doctor told Kelsey that even if I were to defy the odds and survive, I would most certainly spend the rest of my life in a "locked-in state"—a permanent coma.

Kelsey asked to see the CT scan. She had seen many and understood what she was looking at. But she had never looked at one of her husband's brain while he lay in a coma beside her.

What she saw terrified her.

Doctors told her my condition was extremely critical and I would need to be—I must be—moved to The Queen's Medical Center on Oahu. Karma again intruded. Queen's had the only neuroscience ICU on the islands; in fact it was one of very few in the western United States.

A hospital caseworker—whose name was Angel—came in and informed Kelsey that an air ambulance had been called to fly us and a medical team to Honolulu.

Time passed by painfully as the flight was held up by fog.

Frozen by the delay, knowing all too well that I could die at any minute, the banality of small tasks gave some small sense of relief from other, more ominous, thoughts.

Dixie began calling parents and siblings in California and Connecticut, starting just the first drop of what would be an enormous flow of information to the outside world. The first message of what would in the next weeks grow to the hundreds was simple: Get to Hawaii as fast as possible.

Kelsey even called her boss at Kentfield Rehabilitation Hospital near our home in Marin to explain the situation, and to say she wasn't sure when she'd be able to return to work.

There was a question of weight on the small aircraft, which would carry me and my breathing machine, two medics, and Kelsey to Honolulu.

"Are you under one-twenty?" Angel asked.

"One hundred fifteen," she lied.

The flight was eerily beautiful for Kelsey, one last distraction before ugly reality took up permanent residence.

"I'd never seen Hawaii from the air," she would say later. "For some reason I just kept staring out at the spectacular scenery, the waterfalls and the lush tropical landscape, completely taking my mind off the fact that my husband was lying near death just behind me. I suppose I was in a kind of survival mode."

We were met in Honolulu by a medical team and ambulance from Queen's.

The second leg in the most challenging race I ever participated in was about to begin.

Two

QUEEN'S

The inside of an intensive care unit is a study in contrasts. The muted lighting and the calm, deliberate movements of the doctors and nurses offer the illusion of calmness—a façade that provides a sense of security that things are in control and on their way to the right destination. It can be enough to convince those watching that their taut nerves and piercing, nauseating tension are misplaced, that the almost overwhelming fear that is attempting to suffocate them is unwarranted.

For Kelsey and our families, there was the metronomic and reassuring beeping of machines, the small flashing lights, the rhythmic pumps of the ventilator that was keeping me alive. In the background were the quiet, assured conversations, all masking the ever-present blanket of fear that threatened to smother everything. But there was, that first night at Queen's, also sadness and shock and disbelief at what had happened. There was also hope, though, in the mix—hope that I was strong enough to fight my way out. Hope that maybe it wasn't as bad as it seemed to be, hope that maybe the whole thing was just a bad dream.

But it wasn't a bad dream, of course.

In Kona's bright sunshine and comforting breezes a few hours before I pulled off the bike, the biggest decision Kelsey had faced as she hopped from spot to spot following the race was probably what she'd eat at the postrace celebration dinner. We always loved those dinners and the chance they afforded to kick back. Would we share Pinot Gris or maybe a nice Merlot? For a change, maybe have a decadent dessert?

While we were in midair on the way to Honolulu, neurosurgeon Cherylee Chang, my next miracle, received a call to get to the hospital. One of the country's leading neuroscientists, a professor, and director of the Queen's Neuroscience Institute and its stroke center, Dr. Chang listened intently to the information. An athlete had collapsed during the Honu Half. He had been immediately unresponsive, and tests showed a hemorrhage in the brainstem and serious damage. The patient was on the way, she was told, and also had hydrocephalus—extra fluid in the brain caused by a blockage of the usual drainage system by the hemorrhage. Pressure on the patient's brain was increasing dangerously.

The caller told her the patient would need emergency surgery to divert the fluid if he were to survive

Later, Dr. Chang would recall her thoughts as she listened to that phone call.

"I prayed that he would arrive soon enough and kept thinking, 'He's young enough to potentially recover. He's young so the pressure build-up in his brain will be worse for him. Hurry.'"

Dr. Chang rushed to the hospital and was there when we arrived.

What she saw alarmed her.

I was comatose, and Dr. Chang and her staff immediately got to work. I showed signs of severe brainstem injury. I needed a breathing machine. A surgeon placed a drainage catheter to relieve the fluid buildup and to monitor pressure on my brain. Dr. Chang placed catheters to monitor my blood pressure, blood oxygenation, and the removal of carbon dioxide. She quickly gave me medications that could help alleviate the swelling in my brain.

As Kelsey sat stunned, curled up on the floor of the busy intensive care unit waiting for the results of the first tests, she looked up to see Dr. Chang approaching. They were about to have a discussion that no doctor or wife wants to have.

Not unkindly, Dr. Chang told Kelsey the damage was "life-threatening." It was a nice, euphemistic way of telling my shocked wife that I was teetering on the edge, and it was very likely, if the odds played out, I would not make it through the first night. If I had a bit more luck and survived, Dr. Chang told Kelsey, chances were strong I would likely be in a "locked-in" state—severely disabled and nonresponsive, most likely at the mercy of life-supporting technology.

Too much trauma too quickly, it seemed.

"I won't forget how shocked she was to even have this discussion," Dr. Chang recalled later.

Then came the clincher. She asked Kelsey if it came down to it, would I want to be kept alive?

Kelsey and I had talked about such a choice earlier, when such things were a theoretical universe away from the reality she was facing that night. No, I had told her, I would not want to live out my days as a vegetable. Now the stark specter was there, right in her face. Would I hate her if she said, "Keep him alive by any means possible"?

Before such an ominous decision, I had to survive, and at first my chances weren't looking so hot. The first twenty-four to forty-eight hours are crucial. I was in the best place I could be. The decision could wait for a while.

The odd and tauntingly hopeful thing about my brain injury is that over the course of the five weeks I was at Queen's, I woke and spoke and gave my bedside supporters all sorts of false hopes that I would bull my way out. My stay at Queen's was not brief, nor was it one in which I steadily improved. It was an uneven path of peaks and valleys, of glimmers of hope and worrisome setbacks. I was later told that I'd wake up at times and give at least the impression that I had just had a moment of clarity. But these appearances of my old self were teasingly false.

Kelsey would stay by my side for two straight days and nights, fighting off sleep and paralyzing worry.

For the next five weeks, I would alternately provide my family and a wonderful abundance of friends with many opportunities to be both thrilled with my progress and worried that I wouldn't pull through. Such is the drama and reality of brain injuries. It was an up-and-down battle. I'd be on and off a ventilator, I'd have dozens of procedures, I'd fight to pull off the mouthpiece of the ventilator. I'd struggle to get out of bed to the point where they installed netting to save me from further and perhaps fatal injuries from a fall to the floor. I'd have moments of lucidity, flashes of humor, signs that my old self was in there and fighting: thumbs up signs, smiles, and unexpected movements.

So I was told anyway, because I remember nothing of most of that time.

Faced with the nauseating choice of perhaps having to pull the plug, Kelsey called her friend Kiki Silver, an internist, a California neighbor, and part of the triathlon community that would soon envelop us with love and kindness and concern. Kiki's husband, Scott, with whom I trained, and so many others would come through big-time for me later.

"It is way too early to even think about turning off machines," Kiki said. "Dirk is strong, supremely healthy, and determined. Put the thought out of your head."

Even in those first hours, I was responsive to the outside world. When Chris Hauth made it to Honolulu later that night, the first thing he said to me was "Dude, I guess we're not riding tomorrow." I raised my eyebrows. I was listening.

That was the first tease, the initial flash that stirred hopes I'd be fine, that this whole incident would pass fairly quickly. That was the problem, of course, because nothing would pass by quickly. The initial thought that I could be moved back home in a few days to start rehabbing was pummeled regularly by complications and setbacks. Flashes of hope were snuffed out regularly, but hope would always be there, flaring up every time I did something unexpected.

When I first awoke two days later and doctors removed the breathing tube that had been inserted in Kona, I asked, "What was my swim time?" I wanted to know who had won.

I woke briefly and asked for water, not just any water, but San Pellegrino.

I told a joke another time.

I asked for cookies.

But there were cracks in the façade. At one point I woke up and began speaking in clear, perfect German—a language I had not uttered since I was ten.

Eight days into the stay, I was together enough to brush my teeth. I complained about not having had a shower. But these flashes were always temporary.

Even while awake I might shift into talking garbled nonsense. I had trouble tracking with my eyes.

Each time I'd flash a positive sign, Kelsey and my hovering family would think, "He's back. It will be OK."

My loved ones could see the growing frustration eating at me when I would try to talk and nothing came out, when I'd try to get up but couldn't.

The optimism was premature.

But at least the wrenching choice of having to pull the plug was removed for Kelsey by indications that somewhere in there I was fighting and kicking and not about to go gently in that good night, or any night for that matter.

Today, I can still remember pulling off the highway and telling Jimmy Riccatello I thought I was dying. I remember asking Jimmy to tell Kelsey I loved her. I remember Jimmy telling me to close my eyes.

My next clear memory is my mother soft-tossing a Nerf ball at me to see if I could catch it. My mom's toss was more than a month later. Most of what I did at Queen's is lost to me.

In a way, the time in Queen's was much easier on me than it was for our families, who dropped everything and were in Honolulu the next day, comforting Kelsey, pacing the room and trying to will me to get up and say the whole nightmare was a joke—no small feat considering that some made the long trek out from as far away as Connecticut.

Complications did not wait long to set in. The blood that flooded my brainstem was interfering with the network of cavities through which vital fluid flows. I developed hydrocephalus, a blocking of spinal fluid that can be fatal. The large volume of blood that exploded into my skull was making it difficult to even assess the damage. Tissue was beginning to swell. A few days in, I developed pneumonia and a fever. Fluid began to build back up in my head, and surgeons inserted a shunt to drain it. I'd wake briefly then drop back into unconsciousness, where I'd be oblivious to everything, including various attempts to get me to react to pain.

I'd need surgery for deep vein thrombosis. A feeding tube nearly choked me and I went into respiratory distress, which in turn led to Kelsey jumping from my bedside to pound on my chest, pleading with me to breathe again. I had a tracheotomy. I began having panic attacks and would try to pull out the various tubes keeping me alive, what doctors called "bucking the vent." The staff had to tie down my hands to the bed to prevent this. They wrapped the bed with protective netting in case I took a header onto the floor.

Somewhere inside I was alive and ready to move.

By the time Kelsey and I were on board an air ambulance for the flight back to the mainland and home, I would have had multiple procedures. The partial list of daily intrusions reads like the car repair bill no one wants to get: external ventricular drains, shunt revisions, caval filters, cerebral angiograms, central venous catheters, arterial line catheter tracheostomies, multiple CT scans.

After I was discharged, the release papers would catalog the various malfunctions succinctly and without emotion. I had had a midbrain hemorrhage along with an intraventricular hemorrhagic extension. I'd been in a coma and had suffered respiratory failure, tetraplegia, obstructive hydrocephalus, recurrent fever, dysarthria, dysphagia, and diplopia. I'd had a urinary tract infection and deep venous thrombosis.

By the time we headed back home on July 9, I had lost thirty of my 187 pounds. My head was shaved, and those five weeks under the dim lights of the intensive care unit had done nothing for my tan. I was pale as a ghost.

Kelsey would later say that I looked very much like the typical traumatic brain injury patients she had cared for.

All the while, around the country was a small but growing group of friends and loved ones who would reach out in both love and support for Kelsey and my family, who hovered by my bedside as I struggled to settle into at least a vague pattern of regularity.

They became a support team in a way, offering by sheer volume of emails, telephone calls, and letters comfort and love and sympathy. These astounding supporters were all members of the wondrous triathlon community—not just men and women I had raced with and against, but others we didn't even know. We all shared some sort of bond, whatever that might be. The love of competition and the joy of movement and pushing limits, maybe? Whatever it was, the support was astounding. Everyone knew, I guess, that I was in the middle of the race for my life, literally.

An email from Kiki Silver was among the first trickles as word got out—and it shows the illusions of the false hope everyone had during those first days.

After I had raised my eyebrow at Chris Hauth's remark about not training the next day, she wrote:

"This is extraordinary news, nothing short of a small miracle given everything. Kelsey doesn't want to get too excited but we all need to feel the happiness, while still being cautious."

Shortly after the initial note, though, the pattern of hopes raised, then hopes dashed would begin.

Kiki wrote in a follow-up email:

"It is hard to believe that Dirk's amazing progress on Sunday was followed by his less responsiveness the next day. It highlights again how exceedingly fragile the human brain is and even a doctor with high-tech exams, scans, and testing cannot tell how Dirk will be from moment to moment. It can be a series of forward and backward steps. Even the tiniest change in his brain can make him more sleepy, or less able to be roused and lose motor strength. Some patients might, for example, drop their salt level, which can cause comas and seizures."

Much later, at Kentfield Rehabilitation Hospital and at home in Corte Madera, when I was having trouble falling asleep and even more trouble dreaming, I ironically began to recall vividly some bizarre and nightmarish dreams I had at Queen's. Considering the tsunami of medications I was inundated with, including morphine, these dreams were not unexpected. They were eerie side effects of medicine needed to help me control certain bodily functions and stability and keep me free of as much pain as possible. Many were no more than subconscious reactions to what was going on in the outside world while I was out.

They came vividly back to me in California.

In one, I struggled to speak and make myself understood through a slit in my throat, which likely came after my tracheotomy.

While I was on the ventilator, I dreamt that I lived in an underwater world and was forced to swim to swift-moving bubbles to get any life-sustaining oxygen. Each time I'd reach a bubble it would shrink, then burst, and I'd be forced to find another. In reality my lungs were filling with water, which forced me to take shallow and rapid breaths.

In another dream that returned to me later, I was in the basement apartment of friends, trying frantically to stop a stream of water pouring in. Each time I'd plug up one leak, another would spring up elsewhere. It got continually worse, and I was trying to get the attention of my friends upstairs by pulling on what in my dream was some sort of emergency warning cord. In reality, I had been for a time pulling on my feeding tube.

Another even more disturbing dream had me on a conveyor belt passing under a series of sharp and descending blades.

In yet another, and I still haven't figured this one out, I was on a double-decker similar to the iconic London buses. But I was cruising down Broadway in San Francisco past brothels and strip clubs. I couldn't get off. Maybe I should leave that one alone.

While this was going on, the email list seemed to grow exponentially. We were graced with an incredible group of friends, and they, much like Kelsey and our families in Hawaii, faced the same flashes of hope and the same shattering downs.

The first email, from Chris Hauth, went out June 3. I can imagine that Chris was straining at that point to keep his composure and remain cool and unemotional as he spread the first word. His terse note belies his shock at the turn of events earlier in the day:

"Dirk Vlieks of Corte Madera CA was racing on Saturday June 3rd in a triathlon in Kona, Hawaii, and suffered a major bleed in his brain. He was flown immediately to Queen's Hospital in Honolulu Hawaii, and placed in the Neuro-Intensive Care Unit there. Kelsey Vlieks, his wife, was at Dirk's side. We are all hoping and praying for them and will continue to update all of their loved ones with any news."

Chris was back online the next day as I was settling in, if that's the right word, to my new intensive care life at

Queen's. His next email is the first indication that my loved ones were absorbing the fact that there would be many ups and downs in the coming weeks. But his note also shows that early on, the information emerging was informed more by hope than reality:

"Kelsey was at his side the whole way. Here in Honolulu things were up and down for a bit. Brainstems are complicated and we were all extremely concerned—especially since the doctors were telling us the importance of this 24-48 hours. Fluid is being drained from his brain slowly—he has been showing signs of improvement. He had just completed a 'session' of activity where he was asked to give a thumbs up—and he did!"

Chris later added another note to the growing list of correspondents:

"This morning he was more responsive to other demands in his 'sessions'—such as lifting a leg, wiggling a toe, tracking (albeit slowly, but still . . .) with the eyes. These little signs are so important. Then, just thirty minutes ago—while his parents were with him he opened his eyes and responded yes and no to nurses' requests—and did his best Richard Nixon impression—holding up two victory signs with his fingers."

But the hope, as it would be the entire time at Queen's, was tempered by setbacks. Chris added another quick note later:

"He had to be restrained and is back out of consciousness. We are not even close to being out of the woods yet—but he is fighting, like we all know Dirk does—being the Ox we know him as. And he is taking those small steps forward. Just twelve hours ago he was in a completely different state."

One more note that day confirmed the metronomic ups and downs:

"He is writing out letters with his fingers for messages to Kelsey and his family. They had to sedate him since he is using too much energy that he needs for recovery. As we all know Dirk—always trying to push further and harder than he should."

Kiki Silver weighed in on June 5, when the patterns were setting in. The email list had by then grown to hundreds of recipients, many of whom were just hearing the news.

"I am one of Kelsey and Dirk's close friends, I am not sure if you have heard of the recent tragic events. Kelsey asked that I email you so that you would know and could also be kept updated as things unfold.

"Dirk was racing on Saturday in a triathlon and suffered a major bleed in his brain, He was immediately flown to Queen's Hospital in Honolulu and is currently in the neuro-intensive care unit there. Kelsey is there with Dirk's parents and her parents. We are hoping you are praying for them."

As with Chris's quick notes, Kiki's were colored with hope in the early going:

"The next few days will have him hopefully come off the ventilator and working with a speech therapist and doing basic things like sitting up. If they are able to remove the drain and he is stable from neurological and blood pressure standpoint, he'd be able to fly back here soon."

Of course that would not happen and the sentiment was far too premature, since I'd still be at Queen's more than a month later.

But no one knew that at the time, and Kiki's hopes matched everyone else's. Hope springs eternal, I guess, but it does not necessarily match reality.

Kiki added what many were feeling:

"I am so, so optimistic that he is truly on the path to most remarkable recovery. Kels's first glimpse of hope and her happiness today were so good. She kept saying how hopeful she is and how much all of everyone's thoughts, calls, emails, have helped her, Dirk, and her family."

The unimpeachable fact about the whole thing—this "event"—as I look back on it now, almost ten years later, is that I did have a remarkable recovery in the end. It would just take a bit longer than those on the email list and those in the intensive care unit were hoping for.

Chris perhaps summed it up best a few days later:

"Dirk spent most of day three getting tested, although we made some progress yesterday, today is not as good of a day. He was less responsive to the doctors' requests to move and wiggle. He was also not responding at all to family."

Then he catalogued the smorgasbord of conditions that were digging in:

"He does have pneumonia, possible from fluids leaking into the lungs while being unconscious. This is being treated, though given Dirk's other conditions there is much to do."

He continued as reality began to sink in by day four:

"The challenges—today was a frustrating day for Kelsey and family, after yesterday's progress the heart definitely sinks. We all don't want the steps going backwards. But as I have mentioned to Kelsey we all have to realize that we are in this for the long haul.

"Although he gave us hope and relief yesterday, today he brought us back to reality on the severity of the situation."

Then Chris got to the point of the situation:

"I would like to remind all of you praying for Dirk that we still have a lot ahead of us and I hope my communications are properly conveying the challenges and obstacles Dirk must still overcome. I say this not to be negative but to let all of us be sensitive to how long Dirk really needs you all to remain on this 'journey' with him. We are just getting signs of how long and challenging this road will be—with the ups and downs."

Almost a week into our stay at Queen's, a note in the chain from Kelsey's friend Debbie captured the scene:

"I spoke with Kelsey this morning. She sounded exhausted as you can imagine, but trying to stay strong. Lots of family members are over there with her and her mom will be staying indefinitely. They *really* appreciate all of the emails everyone has sent . . . but also noted that they might need to limit this due the overwhelming response."

But again, even a week later, the optimism about the speed of my recovery was still unrealistic.

Kiki wrote:

"The current plan is for Dirk to be transported next Thursday to UCSF, but that is contingent upon his status next week. Here's the status:

"Dirk is weak on his left side, but moving. His speech is a bit garbled but that could be due to the morphine. For the most part he is speaking coherently, albeit with a few hallucinations and random statements. He's had a fever for the past few days, but they are trying to control it.

"He still has the drain in his brain. They are trying to wean him off this, but so far his fever spikes when they try to take it out. There is weakness in his eyes and he has some double vision, but his sense of humor is intact—he even pretended to be a pirate because he wearing a patch over one eye."

Kiki, still speaking several times a day with Kelsey, relayed the next message as my stay at Queen's moved into week two:

"This week in Honolulu had been filled with several hurdles that Dirk has needed to face. Dirk has been able to progress to the point of coming off life support/ventilator and moving all four of his limbs (some more than others). He has been advanced onto a softer diet by a speech pathologist who felt his swallowing was still intact. He seemed, with every day, to be more like "the old Dirk" as Kels said—wanting to go over plans for their backyard shed, giving her the items he needed for her to concoct his salad dressing, etc. But he has appeared to have less of a 'filter'—meaning that he would voice things that normally he would not have; in addition he had periods of being less alert and more confused."

As we moved ever so slowly toward getting back home and starting the real work of rehabilitation, reality was settling in. I had survived. That was the first goal. Next and just as important was getting back to my old self. And as those things settled, the reality that I had not twisted an ankle or torn a knee ligament elicited an emotion I had not permitted myself—sadness.

Self-pity is an emotion I find loathsome. It is an exercise more akin to deep self-absorption, the misguided feeling that as the center of the universe nothing should go wrong. Things did go wrong and I could deal with that—in fact I was dealing with it and would continue.

But sadness, I guess, was inevitable. I was facing the possible loss of a life that had sustained me for so long. I wasn't going to let it control me, but it was there.

Chris caught the sense of it:

"Per Kelsey he seems to be saddened deeply and getting some sense of what is being done to him—she's doing everything she can to keep his spirits up, to give him something to hold onto."

Chis captured the essence of how he felt as he wrote from Coeur d'Alene, where he was preparing for a race he and I had worked so hard for. In a perfect world, I would have been there with him:

"What I will try to do with this email is give us all a bit of perspective on where many of his friends and loved ones will be this weekend, thinking of him, wishing he was here, believing that when we come home Dirk will be in a better state.

"There are so many easy things to say about racing with someone on your mind. It does make you stronger, it does keep you focused and it definitely makes you very grateful for what we have. But to me that would be too easy. Dirk struggling, not because of his current medical situation, but rather his mind is becoming more and more aware of what has happened, what this could mean to his daily life, how this affects his wife and family, what it means for his job, how it impacts his friendships and that for a while he will not be the person he wants to be.

"All this, combined with his incredible sadness of what his wife Kelsey is going through . . . Well, you get the point here.

"So, why am I writing all this? Because we all have many opportunities this coming weekend to live our lives in the way we envision them. Some of us will go to Ironman, others will race Western States, others San Jose Triathlon, Pacific Crest, or even just a weekend of cycling or running with friends.

"Although Dirk can't currently join us on these paths, please take some time to remember how fortunate we are to be able to do what we do in our great community. I know Dirk gets a smile on his face thinking of us all doing what he loves to do. But it also brings sadness that he can't play with us for a while.

"His life is on a different path now."

I was indeed on a different path from that of my constantly moving friends. And the next step was California and Kentfield. When I got there, I would begin the push.

Three

MOTIVATIONS

As the fog began to lift after the ICU at Queen's, the enormity of what hit me wrapped itself around my head. I saw the fear behind the smiles in people's faces, and I was not about to get used to that. I was not about to accept anyone feeling sorry for me. I'd make sure of that. Call it what you might—anger, fear, determination, I'm not entirely sure—but I was not about to adapt to any of that.

While I was growing up, my father's need to move frequently was a karmic match with my own inability to sit still. My family moved a lot when I was young as my father pursued his postgraduate physics research. I could not sit still, even as a two-year-old—crawling, walking, or scrambling over whatever was in front of me.

I was born with a disposition to move. I hated sitting, in fact. Because we moved so much, my brothers and I were always the new kids, always forced to learn the new rules and the new realities of our new homes. This tended to isolate us at first until we settled in. Throw in learning German or French to make friends and you have a recipe for solitary pursuits, which we became very good at—finding things to do while we adapted. We weren't lonely, mind you, because we had our parents and each other. But whenever we moved, we faced some alone time until we settled in.

Looking back at it now, if you were to combine my joy of constant movement with my comfort at spending time alone and you've got the perfect recipe for the creation of a triathlete. I didn't know it at the time, of course, but it did lay down a foundation I would use later. I have always tended to lean to solitary sporting pursuits rather than team efforts. Maybe that's a function of moving so much, or having to make new friends every two years—of adapting to constantly changing realities.

Or maybe that's just me.

But it was a good formula for being pulled at some point into triathlon, for falling in love with it after my first try.

My dislike for sitting still blended well in my early years, when father's postdoctoral research pulled us from Ohio to Canada to Switzerland, Germany, and France before we landed comfortably and permanently in Pleasanton, California, when I was in fourth grade. My father's work was tied to university contracts. When they expired, we moved.

I was the middle child, the second of three boys, sandwiched between my older brother Olaf and younger brother Erik.

We were immersed in new cultures and climates and languages before we had a chance to settle. Moving was a fact of life and it was difficult sometimes with the languages, but I enjoyed it. It was not till later in life that I figured out that because of moving a lot I was also able to acquire many acquaintances and not true friends.

We moved. We adapted. We moved again. It was an early lesson for me in accepting new lives, sometimes one that at first were not entirely palatable. Adapt and move on—I've done both many times now.

As a kid I didn't think that much about our moving around. It was just what the Vlieks family did. But all the while we rarely sat still. We skied, we played soccer, and we joined a European ethos that was not so totally immersed in the couch potato culture of many American kids. That was fine with me.

So by the time we finally settled in Pleasanton, a small city in Alameda County outside San Francisco, the die was cast. I liked solitary sports and I liked to push myself. And the great thing about Pleasanton, a tree-lined, friend-filled place right out of *Leave it to Beaver*, is we stayed. The peripatetic Vliekses finally settled down and settled in one place. It was great. The same schools, same friends, and a chance to settle in without wondering where we'd be moving next.

Pleasanton is the type of small city that lends itself to an easy, comfortable pace. In fact, it was used as the backdrop in the silent film era for *Rebecca of Sunnybrook Farm*, starring Mary Pickford. It was the kind of place where there were farmer's markets every weekend and Christmas parades and Friday night concerts in the park.

Settling in to Pleasanton meant the end of skiing, at least the way we did in Switzerland and Austria, where access to stunning alpine slopes was easy and the sport was as natural as kids playing sandlot baseball in the US. When you live in the San Francisco Bay area, skiing meant long trips. I enjoyed skiing, but again I adapted, or more likely our parents adapted. We would find other pursuits to keep us busy.

My brothers and I had always been competitive. It's what brothers do. Olaf liked tennis, and so Erik and I were given a taste, which pulled me right in. I loved it and couldn't get enough lessons to suit me. Olaf, after challenging me to make the varsity tennis team in high school as a freshman, soon drifted into more cerebral challenges. Erik went for baseball. For me it was tennis and more tennis. When I first started playing, its main appeal, to me anyway, was that it was an introvert's sport, just me alone with the ball, separated by a net from an opponent. Serve, volley, control. No teammates to help, no teammates to blame. I discovered later, as I became more immersed in tennis, that I was wrong about that. But that was later.

When I wasn't playing tennis or taking tennis lessons or thinking about tennis and trying to find a partner to play, I relaxed by collecting things—comics, stamps, baseball cards, coins, rocks, shells—you name it, I had a collection.

My obsession with tennis essentially blinded me to other sports. You'd think at some point, given the number of triathlons I'd compete in later, that I would have at least thought about the track or cross-country or swim teams, but I didn't.

I did compete on the community pool swim team during the summer while growing up, but that wasn't such a big deal, and it was really only something to do when I wasn't playing tennis. Biking? Forget it. I had a paper route and I'd ride around the neighborhood with a canvas bag full of the *Contra Costa Times*, but that was pretty much it for peddling excitement.

I did once get a taste of competitive running, though, a local 5K when I was fifteen. A friend had signed up for it but bagged it right before the start. Since I was standing right next to her when she decided not to run, she impulsively unpinned her bib and gave it to me. I put it on and ran. According to the results, I was the second fastest woman that day. It was an auspicious start to my running career, though the end of my tenure near the top of the women's division.

But tennis was my first love, and I was rarely distracted. Just the smell of a court after a rainstorm will send me back and pump me up, get the adrenaline flowing. I always looked at tennis as a wonderful journey in a way. It's a sport where the destination—winning or losing—doesn't really matter as much as the trip itself—the volleying and the serving and the strategy and psyching out opponents that appealed to me. Being active and staying active, breaking a great and cleansing sweat. I love cleansing sweats.

So I started playing in tournaments, and I begin beating my brothers regularly—and a lot of other kids, as well. I met Olaf's challenge and was playing on the high school varsity as a freshman. I was hooked.

Because I was an introvert, I liked that tennis was a singular pursuit. It's a head game, literally, and I was constantly battling the demons in my own head, serve by serve, game by game, set by set.

I did pretty well as a high school player and by the time my senior year approached I had set my sights on playing in college, of playing for a Division I school. None was more appealing to me than St. Mary's College in nearby Moraga. The Gaels had a good tennis program, and one of my favorite high school teachers had gone there. And I liked the look and feel of the small liberal arts school nestled in the Northern California hills. It had a great Bay-area history. It had some tough entrance requirements, as well, but I met them by doing a year at Cal State Hayward, bringing up my grades to meet St. Mary's rigorous standards and redshirting on the tennis team so I could play four years at St. Mary's. It worked.

I spent my first year at St. Mary's on campus and in the dorms, but for the next three years I settled in to the usual college life of in-town apartments and playing tennis. I had a fairly well-packed schedule, with classes from 8 until 2:30, tennis from 3 to 6, and then work as a waiter and sous-chef at a popular Moraga restaurant. I didn't enjoy the waiting on tables part so much, the hectic pace and the demands to be pleasant and efficient with impatient diners, but I did truly enjoy the cooking, watching how a beautiful and challenging meal comes together. That would later become another of my preoccupations, creating wonderful meals.

By the time I walked back to my apartment after a restaurant shift it would be 1 or 2 a.m., and I knew the whole thing would start again in four hours. Throw in weekends of playing tennis and catching up on homework, and it was not the most conducive schedule for living the relaxing laid-back college life.

But it was fine. I adapted.

I did fairly well in tennis, but I also seemed to refine and improve a growing reputation that I was a "head case" —overreacting in a game that calls for intense but dispassionate and analytical thinking—quick and calm decisions. Being a head case is not a compliment, not a good thing for tennis. I'd more often than not win the first set of a match, calmly and deliberately, but then waver and struggle in the second and third sets as my nerves and head took over.

I did well enough to want to continue to play after St. Mary's, to at least give a shot to seeing how far I could go professionally. My chances for that were slim to none, but I was up for trying anyway. So I played and I traveled: Australia, New Zealand, Brazil, all over the US, just looking for enough wins to spark enough attention to get into a tournament where I might get a few dollars for the efforts—to test how far up I could go.

It never happened. Instead, I was rewarded with sore knees for my efforts. First, there were the years of hammering and pounding that the quick stops and turns tennis demanded, to the point where I began to notice a little soreness after a tough match. But I adapted, I became conscious of making more efficient moves on the court and cutting down on the jarring. This was fine and actually didn't bother me that much. I'd just write it off as the cost of playing.

All that ended when I stepped in a gopher hole on a training run and tore my medial meniscus, the cup of cartilage under the kneecap that provides a smooth base for efficient movement—an essential for the back-and-forth chaos of movement on a tennis court. That injury I could not write off or ignore or adapt to. It hurt like hell. The night after it happened, I couldn't move my leg or bend my knee. By the time I went to bed, my knee had swelled like some sort of mutant grapefruit.

I needed surgery to repair the tear in the meniscus, which went fairly well, though before closing up the surgeon accidently scratched my patella, which would have consequences later. The postsurgery slowness was torture for me. I hated having to sit still for days before I could start rehab. I found it most annoying, as did my friends, who had to deal with my snarkiness while I waited to be able to get up and starting moving again.

But, as my tennis door was closing, another one was opening. Right, it's a cliché right out of a self-improvement book, but in my case it really was true. I needed rehab, of course. My rehab programs called for swimming, biking, weight training, and, eventually, slow and nonpounding running—all designed to give me strength and a full range of motion. Two unintended consequences of that rehab were, first, I realized I liked running, biking, and swimming more than I had known; and, second, I learned I found a certain glow and positive energy from pushing myself. I would push myself to the point of exhaustion, do the swim or weight set or run until I couldn't move. It might seem weird, but I truly enjoyed that place where I found myself after a great workout.

It seemed I had a proclivity for pushing and being able to ignore the pain and tedium that goes along with training. I actually liked it.

One other consequence was that after immersing myself in the rehab, I decided that since I was more or less already doing it, I'd give a triathlon a shot. It appealed to me because, like tennis, it was a solitary pursuit and the endurance side of it, the time and discipline it called for, also drew me in.

So in 1996, with my rehab done and my curiosity about triathlon piqued, I entered my first, an "On Your Marks Tri for Fun" in Pleasanton. It was a short race, designed to gently introduce the curious to the sport. I imagine a few people would never do another, but I would bet many more would want to move on to bigger and longer events. I knew I did. I loved that first race.

I jumped into that first one with no swim goggles, an old pair of running shoes, and a clunky old steel-frame bike I "borrowed" from my unknowing brother. The race was a 400-yard swim, followed by an eleven-mile bike leg, topped off with a 3.1-mile run.

I finished and I was hooked.

I would bet that anyone at the start of their first triathlon thinks about Iron-distance races, mostly about how trying one would be insane. It's probably not unlike someone doing their first mild hill climb imagining making an ascent of Mount Everest. You'd think about it, but that's the extent of it. I certainly did. But somewhere in the back of my mind, Iron distance intrigued me. What would it take?

Three years later, I'd find out.

Ironman was a distance I never thought I would do or could do. I just thought at the time that it was crazy. But a weird thing began to overcome my sensibilities, if I actually had any sensibilities. The more short triathlons I did, and I was getting hooked on them, the more I realized I wanted to try an Ironman.

I needed to learn more about it, about what it took, but I was intrigued. I was also a fairly recent college graduate with a sore knee and the need for a real, full-time job. Full-time jobs can really throw a wrench into training and schedules, and my new job as a computer wonk certainly did. But working full time did not dilute my newfound enthusiasm for triathlons. I adapted. I had managed a pretty crazy work and tennis schedule in school, and I would figure out a way to adapt to this new one, as well. And I did.

My first job was at a paper company, and naturally I hated it, truly disliked the boredom and tediousness of it. But I found a way to squeeze in training by joining a master's swim group and finding time for long early-morning bike rides and runs after work. Weekends were perfect for really doing nothing but focusing on workouts. Once again I adapted.

And something else happened along the way. I met a wonderful group of like-minded people, crazy people who enjoyed torturing themselves as much as I did. It really was a grassroots colony of athletes who loved being outside and loved being fit and training. These were the same people who would rally around me and Kelsey so solidly and lovingly and warmly after the "event."

We weren't one-dimensional automatons. One of my favorite training partners loved to cook, as well, and we'd do long bike rides imagining the astoundingly great meals we'd create and eat at the end of the day. Charles Ehm became a very good friend and took me under his wing, the new inductee into the train-hard, play-hard school of triathlon. I loved it.

Saturday mornings, we'd typically begin hammering an eight-hour training ride with pastries and coffee and end it with massive burritos. Sunday, we'd do what we'd call a 2-2-2—a two-hour swim, two-hour bike ride in the hills, finished off with a two-hour run. This was heads-down, no-lollygagging training, all the time thinking of the five-course meal we'd be eating Sunday night.

I was falling in love with the life.

Later, as we got ready to leave Queen's and head back home for what lay ahead, I knew two things. I would get back to that life, and I would never adapt to anything that demanded I slow down.

Four

TRANSITIONS

Apparently, I was doing exceptionally well.

Within a day, my responses to various stimuli were enough to spark a flurry of hope, tempered maybe just a bit with fear. I was young, and fit, and had always been disciplined and determined. Why would this thing slow me down?

If you were following the string of emails from Kelsey and our friends shortly after I landed at Queen's, you'd think I was on the road to a quick and clean recovery, getting ready to stand, stretch a bit to get loose, and hit the road again.

Hope does that to people. And I suppose if I were awake I'd be thinking and hoping the same thing.

An early email from Kiki Silver, I would imagine, sparked some optimism:

"As Kelsey herself said to me, she wants to be careful not to allow herself to get 'too excited.' It is hard to find the balance between remaining realistic when trying to relay facts to everyone and to be simultaneously optimistic. It is hard to have his amazing progress Sunday to be followed with his less responsiveness yesterday to talking today. It highlights how exceedingly fragile the human brain is and that even the doctors with high tech exams, scans, testing cannot tell you how Dirk is moment to moment. All of these tests help to allow better prognosticating about what will follow, but as yesterday showed it can be a series of forward and backsteps. We cannot allow ourselves to become disheartened when there is a back-step—think of it like kids learning how to walk (once they take their first steps it's hard for parents to see them fall or tumble, but that is the normal path or re-learning and improving, it's not a definite permanent setback."

On June 8, my friend Chris Hauth wrote, "Dirk is talking—somewhat garbled—but talking to Kelsey and family. He has a sense of humor and really wants to get out of bed. Kelsey has been reading him your emails and she wants to say thank you all for your kind words.

"We hope and pray Dirk stays on his current path—which is stable. If he does, we are looking at Dirk coming home sometime soon, maybe next week.

"So, all this said, Dirk is stable. He had a strong fever yesterday but he is feeling better today and it seems we have really taken a few more steps forward in his recovery. It is really fantastic to write 'recovery.' Dirk has given the doctors all the signs for that."

A few days after I had settled in at Queen's, an exhausted Kelsey managed a hopeful note:

"Dirk continues to do well, but as we all know there is a long way to go. He has good cognitive skills, although he gets confused at times, and he has a wonderful sense of humor. He had the place in stitches commenting on the challenge of having to deal with two of me (he still has double vision)."

From the email strings and other hopeful notes, I seemed to be improving so quickly that even in the early days at Queen's, everyone—and that included our relatives who'd dropped everything and had flown out—was thinking of getting me back to California in a matter of days.

On June 11, Kelsey wrote more extensively to the growing email list:

"When and how we can safely move him to SF. (Please let it be soon—I miss home.)"

By then, the ups and downs, the clarity and confusion, the flashes of my old self mixed with complications were wearing everyone down. My parents and brothers and Kelsey's parents and stepparents had all made the long flight out to Honolulu. And unlike the thousands of others who made the same trip, they were not looking to spend days on the beach in the soothing tropical air. They were heading to the tight and fragile emotions of the intensive care unit.

"We need to find out exactly what happened and how to fix it," Kelsey wrote on June 11. "At this point there is too much of a 'jelly mass' at the site of the bleed for us to determine the cause."

As my stay wore on, hope for that miraculous quick recovery was tempered as complications set in. The initial optimism was dampened, wrapped in a wet blanket and smothered by reality. Days stretched to weeks.

On June 17, Debbie wrote about a number of the growing complications, among them problems with the ventilator—my bucking the vent as I struggled to pull out the breathing tube. There were problems with nutrition and the feeding tube and swallowing. There was the drain in my head and not moving anything on my left side, and a blood clot and a urinary tract infection. Such is life in an intensive care unit.

But Debbie wrote of something else, an underlying sub-conscious awareness I seem to have had that something terrible had happened:

"Dirk appears to be more awake today—his eyes opened and he was able to squeeze Kelsey's hand when she asked him if he was hearing her. Per Kelsey he seems to be saddened deeply and be getting some of what is being done to him—she is doing everything she can to keep his spirts up to give him something to hold onto."

It's funny how these things work; how the brain shuts down to protect you from knowing the truth. While our friends were sending out these notes of hope, I was totally out of it, despite my reactions and my humor and movements and comments.

I don't remember a thing about Queen's, of being there, of saying anything or reacting to comments. Not a single thing. Those weeks there are a total blank.

The last thing I remembered was Jimmy Riccitello on race day telling me to lie back on the grass beside the road and to close my eyes and try to relax. The next thing I can recall was waking up strapped to a gurney on the tarmac of the Honolulu International, smelling the jet fuel and hearing raucous airport noise. My mother was tossing a Nerf ball at me to check my reflexes.

That was nearly six weeks after I pulled off my bike on Queen's Highway.

The first words I actually remember saying were to my mom.

"Why are you throwing balls at me?"

That's the first thing I thought about.

By that time, I was thirty pounds lighter and had no idea what had happened, only that the straps on the gurney around my withered arms and legs told something about the tale. At that point I realized I had lost a lot of weight and strength, but that's about it.

Kiki would later note that when she first saw me back in California, I looked like a concentration camp survivor. But waiting to be loaded onto the AirMed ambulance, an ICU with wings, I didn't know how bad I was at that point.

I would learn this later, as I settled into a routine at Kentfield Rehabilitation Hospital in California and consciousness became a more regular visitor. Once I really understood what had happened, I was grateful for the six weeks of not remembering, of not knowing. It was a gift, actually.

Later, I'd remember the nightmares I had at Queen's in those first weeks, when I was on my way to recovery. But the real nightmare for me was about to start—a painful, waking real-life nightmare.

I didn't know that I couldn't walk, eat, or do anything without help. I didn't remember the panic attacks I had at Queen's, or that they had to tie me to the bed. I didn't remember trying to pull out the tubes or bucking the vent.

It started to sink in as the pitch of the AirMed's engines revved for takeoff. What the hell happened? What was going on? We're still in Hawaii? Jesus. What happened at work, and where were my training partners for Coeur d'Alene? What was everyone doing since I pulled off the bike?

It is nothing short of bizarre to blink and lose six weeks.

More than anything, I wondered, what had I put Kelsey and our families and my friends through? What had they been doing the whole time I was out of it? As reality sunk in on the flight back to the mainland, that's what concerned me the most. I was truly sorry for what I must have put people through. I could tell from the way people looked at me when we got back to California, the way they pretended not to notice I looked like a skeleton, I guess. I knew the way I looked shocked the hell out of people.

As my head began to clear, I didn't have much of an idea of what lay ahead, though I knew it was going to be a tough road considering how weak I felt, how hard it was to speak clearly.

That would change, I felt. I'd make them not worry and calm down.

Clinically, as one textbook description put it, "when the patient slowly regains consciousness, he is in a pleasant mood as his view of the world clears. Later, when he begins to recognize the extent of his impairments, he becomes vulnerable to a wide range of debilitating emotions."

That didn't happen and it wouldn't happen, I knew fairly quickly. I didn't have debilitating emotions about anything. I had enough physical debilitations, and I wasn't going to add emotional ones to the pile.

I was upset, to be sure, about a number of things. And as I later settled into my rehab routine, I would begin to hear of the "deficits"—the long list of things I needed to improve or eliminate.

I knew shortly after I returned to reality that I would do right by everyone who had worried.

My first goal was to stay alive. Then I would knock off the deficits one by one—just as I trained, one step at a time.

At that point, freshly conscious and determined, I didn't know about the tumor on my brain stem. No one knew about the tumor. The only concern I had was learning all over again, how to walk and drink and eat and talk.

I knew I'd tap into the whole thing and somehow figure it out. I knew I could somehow draw on my past and my drive and fitness and good health to help. The old Dirk would help this new one.

Don't get me wrong. I was very frustrated. The list of frustrations would grow as I stepped into rehab. The word *frustration* doesn't even begin to express how I felt, from the small things, like sleeping on my favorite right side, which I could no longer do because of the night tremors that would hit with some force. Or being unable to drive a car for a while. I didn't like it, but I'd take a bus. Or not even being able to beat an egg to make an omelet. Then there was the double vision that made even the simplest thing a test. I'd get used to that, as well. I wouldn't like it, but I'd adapt.

And there was losing my dream job and walking like a two-in-the-morning drunk who'd just left he bar after last call.

Yes, those things would bother me. But they would come later.

But I did something that you are not likely to see in any textbooks. First, I had to strip off the negative emotions, the things that would block improvement, the self-pity and the anger. The stroke had happened, and I wasn't going to make it unhappen. I had to get right down to my soul. Then I would improve. Negativity had to go.

The first thing I did very consciously was to develop a very thick skin that allowed me to be able to ignore the frustrations and the stares and the condescension.

By the time I settled into my early days at the Kentfield Rehabilitation Hospital, I was ready to to hit the road and attack whatever lay ahead.

Five

TRAINING

First, a word about the word *discipline*.

Too much is made of it. You read profiles of successful athletes or businessmen and you always note the stress on the guy's "discipline."

He rose early to get into work long before anyone else. Or maybe she was in the pool doing laps before the sun was up. He's a man of steely, unwavering discipline, they will write. Her discipline is what stood out and separated her from her lesser competitors.

I don't buy into that, to tell the truth.

My own feeling on this overrated description is simple. If you like doing something, enjoy doing something—if the benefits of doing that thing, whatever it is, far outweigh the drudgery of doing it—it's not discipline. It is a means to an end. It is just something you do to get to a place you love.

I'll take a break from people saying I was disciplined. It does not take much of an effort for me to do what I love.

Once I got my first taste of triathlon, I joined a club, metaphorically at first anyway. I've always had a group of friends who like to work out together. We didn't have official bylaws. But we did have rules: run with your friends, swim with them, go on long rides, enjoy the camaraderie. Push it. I guess we had dues, too. We paid with the effort we put into training as much as possible. But the rewards of being a member of that unofficial club far outweighed any "discipline" it took to be a member.

We loved it.

Later, when I became totally immersed in triathlon, I actually joined a real club; a team called Kalifornia Kool Stuff, headed and run by former pro triathlete Paul Lundgren. He organized all the workouts, and since I was a glutton for punishment, I did as much as my schedule would allow. There was that small thing about work and making a living, after all.

I loved training. There was no discipline on my part to do what I loved to do. Yes, it was work and took a lot of time. No, it wasn't tedious and no, I did not have any great mental struggle to get out in the early morning as the sun was crawling over the stunning Northern California hills to hit the road with a couple friends. It was beautiful, sublime. I couldn't wait.

It was magic, pure and simple. My training partners were also my social partners, and we did everything together.

It also brought more to me than I invested, which of course is the best sign that you are not wasting your time. Along with the superb physical benefits of long and hard runs, hilly bike rides, and killer pool intervals came another of my goals—happiness and inner peace. That was really what it was all about, since I never was one for collecting winner's trophies.

All that training would pay even greater dividends after the stroke, when everything I had invested came back in spades at a time when I desperately needed it. All those miles and laps were like money in the bank.

So forget the "Dirk was disciplined" story line.

And let's not make too much of how unusual it was, these odd groups of men and women pushing themselves. Take a look at some numbers.

Today there is something like 80,000 people competing for the 2,000 open slots for the Ironman World Championships in Hawaii. More than 30,000 runners did the 2015 Boston Marathon. More than 51,000 runners finished the New York City marathon in 2016. Think about that. 80,000. 30,000. 51,000.

Expand those astonishing numbers by the people who trained for these events but didn't finish. Throw in the number of people on Boylston Street in Boston or in Central Park in New York who watched in wonder as runners went by and said, *Next year.*

What are all these people looking for? Stronger bodies? Stronger minds? Spiritual enlightenment? I think all three of them.

It is all about balance, and I had to learn about that balance. I watched a lot of people get so caught up in the excitement and enthusiasm of entering the world of triathlon that they put the blinders on and became so focused on training they lost sight of everything else.

I was focused on it. But I had my friends and I had Kelsey and travel and food and great companionship. They saved me in a way.

My usual pace is hold the pedal down. When I first realized I wanted to do triathlon, one of the most difficult things for me was to learn how to slow down, how to learn the sport gradually.

You get the idea. We were not alone out there in the Moraga Hills, not some weird group of esthetes cranking out miles. We were part of an astonishing and growing club of people across the country who loved pushing themselves and relishing the benefits.

I will say that being in shape saved my life, or at least it certainly helped. I was in excellent shape as I stood on the starting line in Kailua-Kona. I had spent years setting goals, and preparing myself for various challenges. I had spent years training. There is no way to quantify how much that helped me as I lay in bed at Queen's plugged into machines keeping me alive.

I've heard of people who say that, and I suspect there are many others who think that the human body has only so many heartbeats in a lifetime. Why use them up by accelerating the pace? Why waste them by exercising? You only increase the odds of checking out early.

Of course, that's silly. My workouts increased the odds that I would survive, that I would be able to once again set goals and knock them off one at a time. This time, though, the goals would be a bit different from doing ten hilly miles or draining, breath-stealing intervals on the track. My new goals would be a bit more modest, but they would be goals just the same. Get out of bed. Tie my shoes. Walk home from rehab.

Someone who hasn't had the exhilaration of training and pushing—and of doing it with friends—won't understand. They'd all wonder, what is the point? You're going nowhere, really, and you seem to do it every day. What is wrong with you?

I would beg to differ. It saved me. And those same friends I trained with, and the larger triathlon community who did the same thing, every day, all across the country—they pulled through with me.

That's why I did it.

Ironically, I didn't even finish the first triathlon in Pleasanton. But it was enough of a first taste to send me on my way. The "On Your Marks Tri for Fun" did the trick. I wanted to test the waters for my next athletic pursuit. Tennis was out, at least competitive tennis. My knees couldn't take that anymore. But I still had a bit of a thirst for competition, and my first triathlon quenched it.

After that first race, I knew what I would be doing to take care of the competition and satisfy the itch to keep moving. It's not as if I were overwhelmed with the need to win. It was more of an urge I always had. In tennis I had set goals and fought the voices in my head that told me not to overreact, that told me to stay calm. In the course of a lengthy tennis match that could sometimes be a struggle. In triathlon, with its length and its various stages and disciplines, I had more time to do battle with my head.

I loved the idea of it.

I entered the Tri for Fun cold turkey. I did not run races, race bikes, or swim unless I needed to. While I was strengthening my knees after my tennis career ended, I would take long rides with my friend Rich Au, but it was more for fun than anything else. It certainly wasn't racing.

But as the saying goes, things happen for a reason. After that first triathlon, I was bitten, and those bike rides with Rich took on a new meaning.

In the lexicon of triathlon, that first race in Pleasanton was a "sprint," which is just a euphemism for "short." It is a relative term. Compared to the punishing Ironman, a race that called for a 400-yard swim, followed by an 11-mile bike leg, topped off with a 3.1-mile run is really nothing more than a sprint.

I certainly did not sprint through it, that's for sure. The whole concept of combining those three activities—things I had not really done too much of—was alien to me. But it was somehow intriguing. Was triathlon three separate sports, or did it somehow morph into a single one? How did it work?

I didn't have a clue at first.

The whole point of the Pleasanton race, part of a series to gently introduce competitors to the sport of triathlon, was that it was relatively easy. The run and bike were short and relatively flat—or as flat as things can be in that hilly area. The swim was in a nice, calm lake.

It was not meant to beat entrants down. Those triathlons would come later. But by then, people would know what they were in for.

I didn't know anything that first day, nor did any of the others, I suspect. We were curious.

But once I did my first, I couldn't stop.

That first race started on a clear and crisp morning, the air only like it could be in Northern California on a good day. The sun was threatening to come up as it warmed maybe a hundred or so of us as we stood at the starting line. I was already thinking about what I would do later in the day. I wasn't exactly obsessed with the race or even how I would do. I thought I'd just give it a shot and see what it felt like. It was not as if I felt I was making my next big life choice. There was nothing dramatic about it. I was mildly excited as I watched the others testing their bikes and talking nervously. Since it was a short and inviting race, many of us did not really know what to expect.

I had first heard about triathlons from a Brazilian friend, while I was winding down my tennis career, such as it was. He had talked about triathlons for years, and that had piqued my curiosity. When I heard about the Pleasanton sprint, I thought I would give it a shot.

That first race ended prematurely for me, with a flat tire before I had made it five miles. But that was enough to infect me with the tri-bug. I swore to myself that I would be ready next time. I knew I needed something active to do. And I knew it was not going to be competitive tennis. I enjoyed the variety presented by triathlons—the three-things-in-one opportunity to torture myself. It had a certain amount of appeal, for sure.

Even now, that first race is a pleasant memory that started something that became a long string of pleasant and energizing and wonderful memories. I loved racing and running and swimming. Those thoughts would eventually grow into a vast reservoir of pleasant memories, a lake of positive, energizing hope and strength. Later, when I starting working my way back from the devastation, I would tap into the reservoir. I would draw from it the things that had sustained me in my years of racing. Those memories played a major part in my recovery. I used them to goad myself into moving and meeting my daily goals, whether it was a lap around a field on my mountain bike or walking home instead of talking the bus.

It all started with Pleasanton.

After, given how I always had done things, it was not long before I started thinking about longer distances—and of course, the Mount Everest of triathlon, the Hawaii Ironman.

And so the training began. I was about to start the transition from curious participant to weekend triathlete to serious, totally dedicated yearlong participant. As with everything I did, it was a fairly quick transition.

I knew I wanted to do triathlons. At first, I thought it would be hard to find groups of people to train with and who could teach me. Triathlon was in a grassroots stage at the time, really just starting to catch on with what would become huge groups of participants.

What also appealed to me was the problem-solving aspect, the same thing that had interested me in computers. How did it all blend—the three sports and how to train and balance all that with my daily regular work and social life? That was a challenge and I enjoyed it. It all meshed in an intriguing and weird sort of way. How do I organize the finite number of hours available to me each week and do this?

As I set my sights on the longer races, I fell in with a group of athletes who would goad me and push me. I did the same to them. And I learned a lot—both about talking trash and training. We would rag on one another endlessly and raised the level of insulting to a fine art. We would call it "Talking smack," which required the individual to own it and back it up.

But we also trained like hell.

My training partners were consistent and punctual, which helped me be and train the same way. They also were very good at bringing on the pain, and I did not want to give in, either.

That's why I enjoyed training with others. First and most important, I'm not a solitary guy. I loved the camaraderie and the friendships I developed while I was training. We pushed ourselves and one another. Having the hills of Northern California did not hurt.

I had great like-minded people to train with, guys who taught by example, who showed what it took.

Hey, want to do one hundred miles today?

Sure, no problem.

At first I needed to figure it all out, how to reconcile my regular work day with what I really wanted to do: train and get better. That's the challenge for every serious triathlete.

In a way, there was really no day I could describe as typical, but a week usually went something like this: Monday I'd do a master's swim; Tuesday, a swim and a run; Wednesday, a master's swim in the morning and a group bike ride after work; Thursday, a swim and a run; Friday, a master's swim in the morning and a long run after work.

Saturdays we'd crank it, since we had all day: two hour swim, two-hour-bike ride, and two-hour runs. There was no better way to spend the day.

While I was learning and training, I began to realize I enjoyed biking the best because I would see so much of the beautiful area in one day. Things look different, better, more pronounced when you look at it from the seat of a bike instead of being seated inside a car driving 70 miles an hour. On the other hand, I found swimming boring as hell.

I loved being outdoors, and if I had to run or ride by myself, I had the jaw-dropping beauty of Northern California to keep me company. It was even better doing it with friends. Long rides overlooking the Pacific, trail runs down Mount Tam. You could not beat it.

Or my friends.

I can't say enough about Charlie Ehm, whom I met on a group ride in the Northern California foothills, always a tough one. At the time, I was totally immersed in the triathlon ethic and was gearing up for a killer race in France only a week away. I was still riding 100 miles a day when I should have been tapering. Charlie told me I was crazy, but he didn't lecture me and didn't think I was strange for pushing so close to the race. I appreciated that.

Charlie and I would later do killer training sessions together, running and riding, the whole package. But we would also slow down to fly-fish and to cook astounding meals for our friends.

I met Chris Hauth while training. Chris was an Olympic swimmer, a gifted all-around athlete, and, like me, a glutton for punishment, and that pushed us to the edge. We once became intrigued by skate-skiing and exhausted ourselves learning how to perfect the awkward technique. And I'm so indebted to Chris, who did so much after my stroke.

Steve "Scuba" Holmes was another guy I met through triathlon. And like so many other friends I met along the way, ours was not one-dimensional friendship. In addition to pushing ourselves on long rides, we were both into computers, comic books, good movies, and strong coffee.

I do have to make clear that I've always been pulled by physical challenges. At one point I had read about a trail run— an actual organized race—from base camp on Mount Everest. It sounded insane. It sounded great. I wanted to do that and probably would have, but life intervened and I never got it together. I think it would have been fun.

It hurts, therefore it is fun. I always wanted to do more. I relished pushing the envelope. So did my friends.

As my training progressed, I learned there was more to triathlon than simply putting in miles. Everyone has a strong suit, and a weak suit, no matter how many hours they put in. Triathlon is a great sport because you will always be trying to get better at something. Success is always relative. It keeps you motivated, and triathlon offers many different ways to achieve success.

When I first started, I had one simple plan in my head—swim like a swimmer, bike like a biker, and run like a runner. That meant early morning or late evening master's swim classes to work on endurance and technique. To improve my running, I found a group that would have track workouts. I found a lunchtime bike group, and we'd push through noontime rides up the peninsula or around the East Bay. Weekends, I'd hook up with riders for painful ride around San Anselmo.

I found the learning fun and the training exciting.

In a way, triathlon is a lonely sport. But it is not a sport of loners. We trained together and encouraged one another. We did it together. When we were done for the day, we'd kick back, eat burritos, have a glass of good California wine. Soak it all in.

One of the most important things I had to learn was about how to pace myself. Early on I had to take days off because I was too sore and stiff to walk down the stairs. I learned pretty quickly the stuff I did to induce those days off was simply dumb due to bad training. I learned how not to do that to myself. I learned how to pace myself so I would start every workout with energy, not to just have barely enough in the tank to make it through the run or the ride or the swim—whatever we had planned for the day.

For a break, I'd play some tennis. Just for kicks, mostly. It certainly was not the center of my sporting life anymore. Triathlon and endurance racing had taken its place. I knew if I started getting intense about my tennis, my knees would once again be too shot to do anything. Triathlon was relativly gentle on my knees, since the biking and running were rhythmic and not jarring. Swimming did nothing to harm them.

I trained to get better, not to win. In fact, the prospect of winning a race never entered my mind. Racing smart was my end goal. I was not one to enter the same race every year. A lot of competitors did that to beat their previous year's time. There were so many races in so many interesting places, I wanted to try them all. I knew how to gauge my results—if I had done well—just by how I felt. I did not need to beat my old times.

For years I would do short races such as the Monterey Challenge, Sandman, Uvas Reservoir Triathlon, and many others, some of which aren't even around anymore. I raced at some very cool places and I met some very cool people. I accumulated friends and experiences with each new race.

By 1998, it dawned on me I wanted to do longer races. I had done the Vineman Half Ironman a few times, and I wanted to step up my game by doing the full Ironman. I did, finished it, and loved it. I was totally pulled in.

I began to expand and to do longer races in interesting places. That was part of the pull. I raced in the Tahoe Challenge, Santa Barbara Triathlon, Monterey Bay Challenge, the ITU Nice, in France, and the Coeur d'Alene Ironman.

I never had a bad race, never experienced a moment of doubt over the time I spent dong this crazy stuff all over the country.

I was totally in. And I was exceptionally happy to be there.

Six

THE ROAD BACK HOME

I'll take a wild guess and say that I doubt the cigar-smoking, brandy-swilling Winston Churchill spent a lot of time working out. But he did have something to say about getting knocked down and springing back up that I can identify with:

"Success consists of going from one failure to the next without loss of enthusiasm."

I didn't fail, of course; my body did. I had to deal with it just the same.

When I took my first steps toward recovery—literally and emotionally—I was not blessed with a blinding-light epiphany.

There was not a single clear flash that illuminated the path ahead. When I got to rehab, I knew I would never have the same body again. I shed as much frustration about that cold fact as I could. Instead, I began to focus on one thing: if I were going to have to deal with a new body, I was going to make absolutely sure it was a strong one.

I wanted to come back as close as I could to my old life. If I couldn't get there, I wanted at least to be in the neighborhood.

Recently, I spoke with a woman who is a fourth grade teacher, and what she said made sense to me:

"I work with some kids who are unable to do some simple functions, like run and play. They see the other kids do this, and they try harder so they can play as well. They want to be included."

I wanted to play again, to walk and run and hit my stride again. I felt that primal urge we all have to regain our place in the herd.

That was my mission at Kentfield Rehabilitation Hospital, the small, comfortable facility tucked into a tight sunny Northern California neighborhood on Sir Francis Drake Boulevard. It was not a spa, not some place where patients lay back in the sun's warm embrace and respond to the gentle prodding of physical therapists.

I was not there to recuperate from a broken leg or a bruised ego or whatever malaise drives people to rehab. I wasn't there to rest and renourish and shake off the bumps and bruises of an unfortunate mishap like a skiing accident or a bad hit in a touch football game with the boys.

I was there to get my life back at its most basic level. I was starting at square one. I worked hard, as hard as I ever worked. I wanted to be out of there and home as quickly as I could. I would walk, then I would run. That was how I felt.

My time at Kentfield was a serious challenge, a rawness that intervened with what had been a smooth life, where through my own hard work and planning everything was meshing in great synchronous joy. The stroke had rudely and indelibly changed that on a number of levels. First, of course, I had to accept the fact that I was there in the first place, that I needed some serious help.

I had spent six weeks semiconscious in Hawaii, which was not a bad state of mind considering what had happened. At Kentfield, I no longer had the luxury of being out of it. My stroke and its ravages were beginning to sink in. I was awake. And I was aware that I was not in a good position.

This is not meant as some hand-wringing lament at my misfortune. More than anything, I was alive, and by all accounts damn lucky to be. I knew that. And I know that now. I did not feel sorry for myself or ever at any point succumb to bitterness or self-pity.

It had happened and I could not change it. I would deal with it.

When I arrived at Kentfield, I couldn't walk. I could barely get out of bed. I had lost thirty pounds. I could not express myself clearly, and I needed help to even do something as simple as taking a drink of water. My vision was blurred and my entire left side shaky at best.

It was not a good thing.

I did not want to be there, and I quickly—immediately—made it my mission to get out as soon as I could. And never return.

Even in the marketing language of its brochure, Kentfield makes it clear it is not a summer camp.

"Kentfield Hospital is a licensed acute care hospital specializing in the care of complex medical and rehabilitation patients, who may require extended stays to achieve the best recovery possible. Located just north of the Golden Gate Bridge in a tranquil wooded setting in the heart of Marin County, our 60-bed facility has over 30 years' experience providing outstanding patient care."

By the time I left Kentfield, the staff called me a poster boy for their program. It was not exactly like crossing the finish line in Hawaii, but I'll take that as a compliment. By the time I walked into my front door at home for good on August 25, I felt solid and confident I had done all I could, maybe even more.

When I first arrived at Kentfield, I was faced with learning like a two-year-old how to do things all over again— to walk and eat and sip and talk. It was pretty basic stuff, but that was what the stroke had done to me. Within six weeks, working with my physical therapist Hans Gouwens and others, I learned how to walk and talk and eat again—the primal basics, I guess, like a two-year-old suddenly thrust into an accelerated "here's how you live" program. I graduated with honors, though. I would come home with Kelsey on August 19, just in time to celebrate our second anniversary. My friend Charlie Ehm cooked us a five-course meal.

My time at Kentfield was a mixture of frustration, hope, and challenge. It was trying and emotionally draining, to say the least. But like anything I had ever done, I had a goal and I set my sights on it. It was not all smooth sailing and gusts of rosy happiness. It was hard.

But I did have one thought that I woke up with every single day, ready to hit the bricks again. It became my mantra. If I were inclined to tattoos, I'd have it inked on my forehead, maybe in bright neon letters.

"Every day is a gift."

Our first day at Kentfield had been eagerly awaited by our friends and family who had been watching the drama unfold from a distance. They all had wanted to help in some way as soon as they heard but couldn't while we were in Hawaii.

During my stay at Kentfield I was surrounded by those friends—those wonderful supportive, loving friends. In fact, when I think about it, I rarely had a moment alone, and that, of course, was nothing short of wonderful. I didn't need to be alone. I didn't want, really, to be alone too much. I needed to keep occupied so I would not overly reflect on what had happened.

For our friends, there was a practical, almost dryly pedestrian side to the plans, and our friend Jeri Howland made that clear right from the start:

"Dirk and Kelsey arrived in Kentfield at about 1 p.m. and now Kelsey is getting settled in her lovely home she has missed so much for almost five weeks. She looks great and has such a strong and positive mindset. There is a lot for her to adjust to right now. So in terms of food support, for the moment she would really like some privacy and time to adjust to being home and figuring out what she needs.

"When she is ready I will send out a calendar so that anyone who wants to bring food can do so in an organized and appropriate fashion.

"What she wants to eat and have in the fridge: Kelsey is a fairly particular eater—and if she isn't home alone there is likely to be one or two members of her family staying at the house which means large pans of lasagna will be too much."

As I said, right down to the barest of details.

We had left Queen's and flown to the mainland on an AirMed ambulance with me looking like some sort of disaster survivor and still under intense medical supervision. When I first arrived at Kentfield, I was labeled "max assistance." I could not sit up without help.

My physical therapist at Kentfield was a friend and training partner, Hans Gouwens—which was a blessing in more ways than one. Hans knew me, knew how I trained, and how I loved to push it. He did not spare me, and for that I am eternally grateful. Before my unintended stay at Kentfield, Kelsey and I would often drop by for dinner with Hans and his family.

It was good to have a familiar face with therapy. We worked well together, and I was not going to give an inch to him or myself.

Shortly after I arrived, Hans joined the email chain. His first note was optimistic:

"Kelsey and Dirk are back in Marin. I have seen Dirk for a few days now at Kentfield Rehabilitation Hospital. On Monday he took his first steps in five weeks and yesterday he walked 2 X 75 feet with moderate assistance. He has made some great progress in just a few days, but he still has a long road of rehab ahead of him. However, he is strong, motivated, and eager to climb out of bed when he has the chance. He does get fatigued easily and needs lots of rest in between his therapy sessions."

Chris Hauth was able to fill in some other details right after I got there, as well:

"Dirk is still quite weak and, as many of you can imagine, in a very vulnerable situation. Therefore visits might be somewhat awkward for him as well as draining."

I guess Chris was reminding people that I had not just returned from a relaxing surfing trip to the islands. My head was still partially shaved from various intrusions into my skull. I looked, as Kiki has said, like a concentration camp survivor, rail thin and pale as a ghost.

Chris's note emphasized that:

"Dirk has lost a significant amount of weight, still has a trach and is limited in his facial expressions—for these and a few more reasons, I would like us to wait a few more days until Dirk has made more progress. Lastly—he also cannot speak yet, and the frustration of not being able to communicate with his visitors can also get overwhelming."

There is the one word, the one emotion—frustration—that I did not care to invest in. It was there for sure, and I felt it. But I would fight to repel that stark and useless emotion as hard as I could. I did not need to go there.

For my friends and family who were with me in Hawaii and for those watching from a distance, the whole experience was certainly a yo-yo of emotions. At first hoping I would live, then perhaps hoping it was minor and that I'd be up in a few days, and then slowly letting the reality of it all sink in.

Chris, who knew me as well as anyone, who knew how to push me, began helping Hans with sessions.

After I was at Kentfield a few days, he wrote that I was "doing much better":

"I did the morning session of PT with him yesterday and was also really encouraged in seeing how well he is doing, how determined he is and I am confident in his improvement over the next few weeks to a point where we will be able to have the Dirk back we all know well."

And through it all, Kelsey forged ahead as only she can.

Chris wrote:

"Kelsey is still quite exhausted and overwhelmed from the last five weeks and now the dramatic change from intensive care to a rehab center. She is still spending a lot of hours with Dirk and therefore her energy is devoted to his improvement. Shouldn't be long before we can all go see him, please be patient for a bit more."

Kelsey and I both wanted to get out of Kentfield as quickly as possible. But I think we were also like many people waking up from a bad dream, shaking off the cobwebs, and hoping things would be back to normal. But we couldn't quite do it. By the time we were fully awake, we knew it wasn't a dream and we knew we had to deal with it, all of it. It was not going away. We knew we needed to just get going, deal with it, and move on.

And so I did. Everything I did was to push myself, force myself back to normal. That was my goal and my motivation that I started immediately.

While Kelsey settled back into the home we had left so blissfully six weeks before for what we had thought was a short jaunt to Hawaii and a race, I went at it as hard as I could.

Lying in bed for five weeks can in itself wreak havoc on muscles, not matter how toned they are. They atrophy quickly. Add to the mix the fact that I'd been poked and prodded and intubated and tube-fed and in and out of consciousness, so I was not in the best of shape my first morning at Kentfield. Trying to get out of bed was as challenging to me as any Ironman.

Very quickly I went at it.

Within a few days I could dress myself. I did not miss the open-backed hospital gown that had been my uniform for what felt like forever. It felt good to finally have some cover for my backside. Those gowns might be convenient for hospital staffs, but they do not inspire public confidence unless you're an exhibitionist.

Getting dressed soon included putting on my sport ASICS DS trainers, a sort of cult shoe for hardcore runners. Those shoes would not be accumulating the mileage I would normally be putting on them, but putting them on, and slowly and painstakingly tying them, was a major milestone.

My battle each day became somehow overcoming what the physical therapists euphemistically called my "deficits"—just a few small things—like regaining my strength, my endurance, my balance and coordination, and speaking. Also, learning how to eat and drink without massive spillage.

My schedule was ambitious, and I was ready for it. Six thirty-minute sessions each day, with each session focusing on one deficit.

In between those sessions a stream of people dropped by, Steve "Scuba" Holmes, Chris, guys I trained with, men and women I raced with, coworkers, neighbors, and of course family, my brothers and parents and Kelsey's family. It was nonstop, and it was gratifying and beautiful.

Scuba would visit regularly and bring me a cup a coffee and would help me shave in the morning. Then I would head off to my first chore of the day, emptying the dishwasher. Eating was a bit of a chore, as well, for the most part because the food was soft and, as far as I was concerned, very bland. It had to be, of course, because I could not chew. It was what they called a "mechanical" diet. Quite unappetizing, I must say. I faced some other issues, as well. Remembering the simplest things was difficult, and my trach—a tube inserted to help me breathe—was not exactly fun.

I also realized that I would need glasses. It was impossible to see clearly without them. Everything came at me in an almost nauseating double vision.

The final annoyance—it was mortifying to me, to tell the truth—was getting locked into bed at night and not being able to get up to use the bathroom. Falling would have presented a complication I did not need at the time. The Kentfield staff decided to make what they called a tent that prevented me from venturing a midnight stroll to the bathroom and maybe taking a massive header into the hard floor.

"He is not safe to go alone and a fall is the last thing we needed to add to our curve balls," Kelsey wrote to the email list.

I was OK with all of that, though. They were just irritations I would have to put behind me. The faster the better as far as I was concerned.

The realization that life was going to be different was setting in. My PT would work with my left-sided weakness, and no matter the exercise, I would always do one more, I was not satisfied with just getting by. I had PT, OT, SP, and other acronyms daily.

In the rare moments when the quiet settled in, I could count on Kelsey to think of something else to do to keep me occupied. I had no time alone, and that was good.

Kelsey expressed the reality of the situation succinctly when she wrote two weeks after I was brought in, "Cognitively, Dirk is with us—thank God."

Of course that was wonderful news. But as she continued her note, the kicker settled in, the cobwebs were off and clear, and our heads were beginning to wrap around the situation, to absorb the reality of what we faced:

"Dirk is becoming more and more aware of what happened and the ramifications. He expresses his emotions well and told me how sad he is for me that this happened. So, we talk a lot about how were are a team and we're going to get through this together and we are better because of it. Through all of this, though, Dirk's personality is shining through; actually, I think he's developed quite a sense of humor. He laughs, cracks jokes, flirts with the elderly ladies, and waves to everyone he sees."

I wanted to go home. I wanted to wake and shake my head and be washed by the immense relief that the whole thing was a bad, tortured dream. Both Kelsey and I both wanted that. I told Kelsey that every day.

But the reality was that was not going to happen right away.

Kelsey realized that first. She knew that Kentfield was the best place for me to be, to maximize my care and efforts so that when I did actually get home, the readjustment would not be severe, that I would be safe both physically and cognitively.

For one thing, I was not exactly safety-conscious. Kelsey accepted that as part of the damage done. I might disagree with that. I had never been safety-conscious. I was not one for gentle steps. I rode in traffic. I took downhill curves on the bike as fast as I could. I loved blasting through the surf.

Instead, now it wasn't steep roads or bashing waves, it was getting out of bed.

By two weeks in, I had buoyed everyone by what Kelsey called "slow and steady" progress:

"He walked 150 feet this week, with assistance, which was really exciting. He wobbles but his balance reactions are improving. He is feeding himself 80 percent of the time and is enjoying every sweet he can get his hands on."

Kelsey, ever health-conscious and meticulous about what we ate, was putting a damper on that, though:

"Dirk's roommate has a sweets drawer and I was denying him chocolate, as was his brother. Well, we stepped out of the room for a few minutes and he coerced a nurse into getting him the chocolate—I couldn't believe my eyes. He was very proud of himself."

While I was attending to the various debris left by the stroke—my balance, memory, speech, and endurance—there was another constant we had to deal with.

I could not see straight. I would wake up each morning hoping it would not start again, but when I opened my eyes I saw everything in twos. And by the end of the day, when I was tired from my various exertions, everything was pretty much a blur, and I could not look up and down without become very dizzy. This did not help my balance problem.

Kelsey, as only she could, made light of it, trying to convince me that seeing two of her was an amazing gift. I agreed, but it was still annoying.

A neuroophthalmologist gave me a series of Botox injections, three in my right eye and one in my left. The theory was that the injections would relax the muscles surrounding my eyes and even out what he called my "disconjugate gaze."

These injections, the doctor said, would take ten to twelve days to begin working, but the next day I woke up and swore I could see better. Maybe I was turning the corner, I thought.

I began to understand that recovery was not linear. It was not, in the simplest of terms, one step in front of the other toward a goal. There were things going on all over the place, some forward and positive, some backward. Some things did not change at all, for better or worse. But in general, things did seem to be moving in the right direction.

Take the clots, for example. About a week after I settled in at Kentfield, a scan showed I had developed blood clotting in my legs. So it was off to Marin General Hospital to have a filter placed in my inferior vena cava. It was supposedly a relatively benign procedure, but it had larger implications. If I continued to clot, I'd be on blood thinners for the rest of my life. Not an enticing thought.

At the end of July, with my eyes feeling a bit better, another scan showed that the clots had disappeared. We were moving ahead.

But things never went as planned. In the relatively simple procedure to remove the filter, the surgeon nicked my femoral artery, which then required an additional five hours lying flat on my back—I guess to make sure I didn't erupt—until doctors were certain it was safe for me to return to Kentfield.

Things were heading mostly in the right direction, though. We were allowed to make a quick stop at home for a few hours. It was comforting to see my cats again, and to just get a glimpse of our past life—to be able to soak in the wonderfulness of it all.

August awaited, and with it my gradual but positive improvement, finally; and as things settled down, we needed to find out what had caused this whole thing in the first place. What exactly had happed to me on the Queen K Highway?

Kelsey wrote to the growing number of friends and supporters:

"Next week is a big week. Monday we are going to UCSF for a follow-up MRI. Then we'll return for an appointment to discuss the results and the next steps. We still don't know why this happened and we may never know, but it is important that we search for some answers, if they are to be found."

We would find the answer. And with that came new tensions, a new and near-electric fear, and a glimmer of hope.

It all depended on how much of a chance we wanted to take with the rest of my life.

Seven

THE RAZOR'S EDGE

It hovered over us like a malevolent ghost. We knew it was there, drifting ominously, wrapped around every single thing we did, day and night.

What, exactly, had happened out there on the Queen K Highway, and what were we going to do about it?

No matter what positive event buoyed us, and there were plenty, that cloud hung above us and we couldn't shake it, though Kelsey and I dealt with it in different ways.

There was not one single day, probably not any single moment, when we were not thinking about it. It was a dangerous dance, being happy with the progress I was making while worrying about surgeons having to probe inside my brain and perhaps disrupt things all over again.

I did know and appreciate one thing, though. At least I was dancing.

I got out of Kentfield, which I had grown to appreciate in an odd sort of way. But I was tiring of its sterility and regularity and lack of spontaneity. The routine at Kentfield was wearing me down emotionally. I was tiring of the constant reminders that I was not normal. I was sick of hospital settings and therapists. I was ready to go home and work from there.

After weeks of hard work and pushing at Kentfield, I won one battle. I went home on August 25. But three weeks after I had begun to savor the comforts of being home, I would be back in the hospital, undergoing surgery, and then once more back in an ICU while I recovered.

But I would be in that recovery room because I wanted to be, because Kelsey and I had taken a nervous, taut, and calculated risk that the surgery would remove that cloud, that after that I would be free to work as hard as I could to get my life back.

The surgery would be worth it, despite the enormous risk and the knowledge that in many ways I'd be starting all over again, almost from square one. But this time, instead of the ambush on Queen K Highway, I would have planned and welcomed the intrusion. And this time, I knew that all the work I had been doing at Kentfield was like money in the bank, an investment that had prepared my body for another assault. That's why I continued to work hard at home to get ready for the surgery that would remove the growth that sparked the whole nightmare.

Or at least we hoped.

But it was back to that question: What caused this whole nightmare in the first place? It had hung so heavily over Kelsey and me while I was at Kentfield. As I worked my way through the days there, the questions and worries and decision making glared at us constantly. It would not go away. If the surgery went awry, or if any number of very real complications set in, I'd be in bigger trouble than I already was.

It was not a comforting thought.

But on the other side of that cloud was the hope that if everything went well, we'd never have to worry about it again.

The stoic and always-resilient Kelsey would break occasionally. She is by nature an optimist and a strong woman, but her strength would crack at times and she would let it get to her, admitting to private tears and frustration. On the other hand, I kept up my appearances. I kept my fears to myself. As I look back on it now, ten years later from a far different perspective, I even kept my fears from myself.

The subconscious mind is powerful. By definition it is mysterious and uncontrollable. The truth of the matter is, while I acted the part of the energetic and enthusiastic patient at Kentfield, I was having nightmares. The sleeping problems I still have occasionally even today began at Kentfield. I could not sleep on my back. I could not sleep in certain positions. I could not sleep well at all. Something was going on. As I tried to sleep, my subconscious mind was taking over, and it manifested itself in neck and back pain and all the things that tension and inner turmoil provide.

At Kentfield, I internalized the stress. By all appearances, if the Kentfield therapists and staff and my many visitors looked, they would have seen the old determined Dirk, working in his usual diligent and carefree manner. But at night, when I was asleep, or at least half asleep, my mind took over, and I would twist and toss and churn.

It was painful. It was my worried mind, saying all was not well. Inwardly I was a mess. We even tried massages, thinking that would release whatever tensions seemed to be building. But massages could not reach my subconscious mind.

On the surface things appeared to be going well as I worked my way through the rigors of Kentfield, and in many ways they were. But there was always in the background, the gatecrasher who would not go away while everyone else at the party tried to ignore the obnoxious and ill-mannered boor in the center of the room.

Would it happen again?

By August 1, I was doing well enough at Kentfield for Kelsey to write to a growing number of friends and supporters on the email list:

"Not surprisingly Dirk has continued to do well in rehab. He walked to Ross and back on the bike path, which is a little over a quarter mile away, with minimal assistance. His balance is slowly improving and fortunately his balance reactions are improving even faster. That means he is starting to catch himself when he begins to fall."

My chore list and my first steps back into the real world were also beginning.

"He has also been working in the kitchen loading and unloading the dishes. On Monday he is going to make himself a smoothie for breakfast; he's really excited to get back in the kitchen."

But that was just on the surface.

I was not exactly ecstatic about being able to accomplish something as pedestrian as unloading a dishwasher. Don't get me wrong, I was happy for every single improvement, every small gift that showed I was coming out of it. But I was impatient for something more challenging, more creative, more real. I did not want to be applauded for doing something a child could do.

There was much turbulence going on underneath it all. Beneath that calm and happy surface, my mind and brain was roiling with tension. My subconscious mind was alert and working—and it was injecting some unsettled feelings I did not want and I could control.

Why had this happened?

Kelsey could write upbeat notes to our friends:

"Dirk's speech improves daily. We are working on intonation and facial expressions."

"He keeps us all laughing during speech sessions because he says some of the most random, funny comments. He makes himself laugh a lot, which is wonderful."

But beneath it all there were rough spots, irritating little burrs that would remind us that I wasn't at Kentfield because I fell off my bike and scraped my knees.

"Dirk's eyesight is still an issue. He continues to have double vision. His vision is definitely improving and his eyes are becoming more level, but it's frustrating for him."

"We were told by the doctor yesterday that it may take a year for his eyes to heal and if they don't there are surgical options. This means I will be doing all the driving for some time—oh boy. I think we will be sticking to Marin County."

That was all fine, believe me. I was alive and up and moving and beginning to crack the shell that had kept me off the streets for the last two months. I was, more than anything, grateful.

But we had to know and wanted to know what was wrong. I was fine with learning what had caused the problem. I was not afraid. In fact, I needed and wanted to find out what happened just so I could move on.

So I became the poster boy for Kentfield, its great success story. I was challenged, and of course I loved being challenged. In a way I looked at it as simply another race. I joked, I flirted and made people laugh, and I tried to comfort Kelsey, to make her briefly forget where we were and why. She had gone to Hawaii to watch a race and soak up some sun, to take in the sweet eucalyptus-scented air of Maui. Now she was taking in the Lysol-ridden air of Kentfield wondering what had happened. It seemed unfair, and I wanted to relieve her of the stress.

I certainly looked at my time at Kentfield as a gift. I was lucky it happened where it did, on the road, surrounded by people and with medical staff nearby. I did not want to waste that gift, and I didn't. I worked hard to get out as quickly as I could to enjoy the even more sumptuous gift of being home. That's where I wanted to be.

So with the unanswered question hovering over us while we waited for tests and analyses and judgments, I worked madly. I did what I was told to do by Hans and my other therapists. I gained back fifteen pounds. I coveted the rewards of all the gummy bears I could cadge from the sympathetic staff and my roommate's candy drawer.

My eyes continued to improve, slowly anyway. I finally got to the point where I could control their movement, and I was able to tell Kelsey almost triumphantly that the two of her I always saw were beginning to move closer together. I could begin to track people moving across the room and follow them from side to side. I could move my eyes up and down without losing focus, which in the early days had done nothing but produce chaos and dizziness.

My appetite, never a weak point, improved every day. I had been on what they called a "mechanical diet": no steak, lettuce,

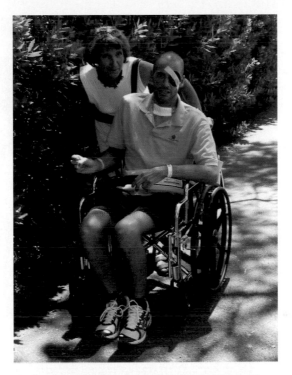

With my mom in August 2006. I had joked about the patch, but I was serious when I first got to Kentfield. *Photo by Kelsey Vlieks.*

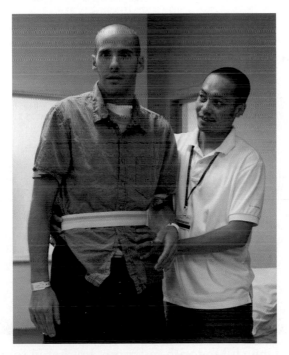

When I got to Kentfield, I could not stand, so this was progress. *Photo by Kelsey Vlieks.*

On the bike path by our house, with Kelsey watching my balance. It was great to be outside. *Photo by Ute Vlieks.*

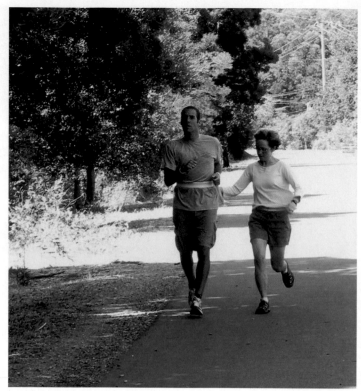

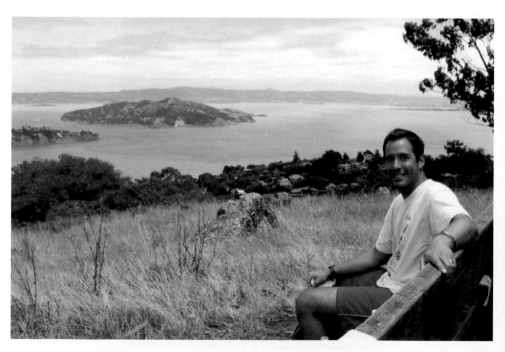

I didn't sit often while hiking with my mom, but here I took a break in the hills above Sausalito. *Photo by Ute Vlieks.*

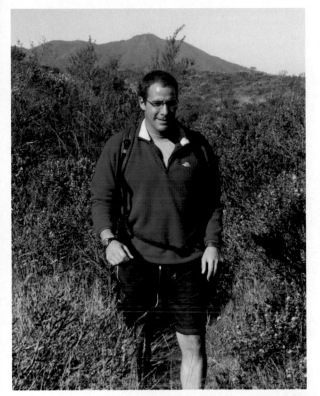

Balance and endurance work, April 2007. No better place to do it than the California hills. *Photo by Ute Vlieks.*

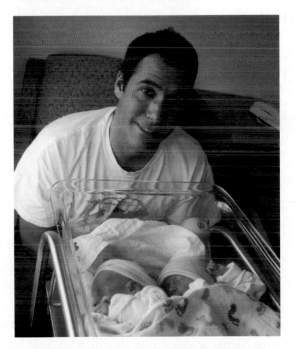

Proud Papa. With Anna and Ellie Vlieks shortly after their arrival at Marin General Hospital in 2008. *Photo by Ute Vlieks.*

With Ellie at the hospital. *Photo by Ute Vlieks.*

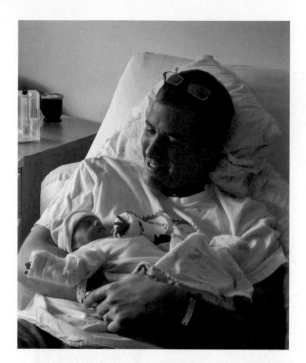

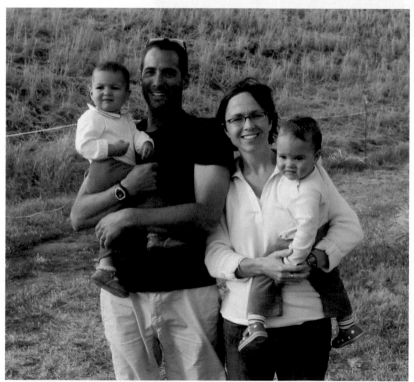

Our growing family. With Kelsey and the girls at my parents' house in Livermore in 2010. *Photo by Ute Vlieks.*

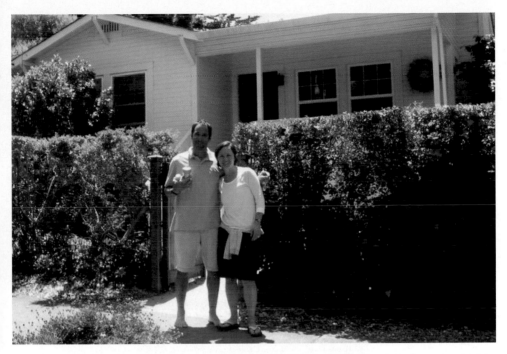

California comfort. In front of our old house in Corte Madera in 2010. Getting back there was a major goal. *Photo by Ute Vlieks.*

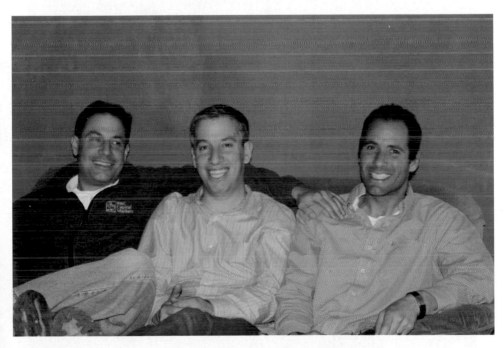

The Vlieks Brothers at rest. With Erik, left, and Olaf at our parents' house in Livermore in January 2011. *Photo by Ute Vlieks.*

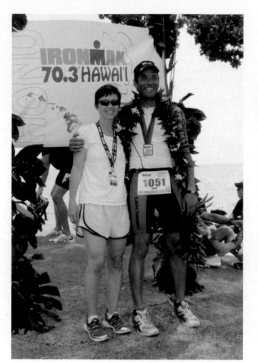

Relief. My DNF had irked me for some time. Smiling at the finish of the Honu Half Ironman on the Big Island, with Kelsey, June 2011. *Photo by Ute Vlieks.*

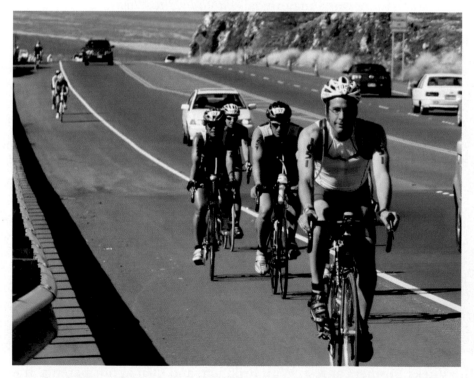

On the bike and headed for some closure. I barely blinked after I passed the spot where it all started. *Photo by Kelsey Vlieks.*

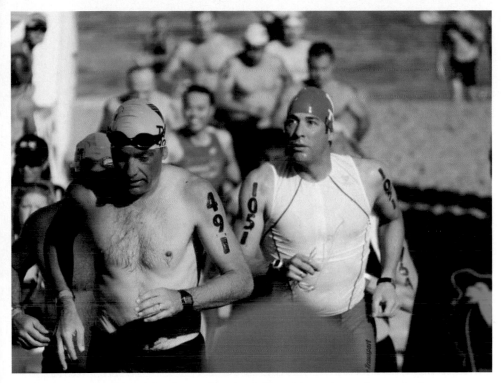

Out of the water and looking for my bike. *Photo by Kelsey Vlieks.*

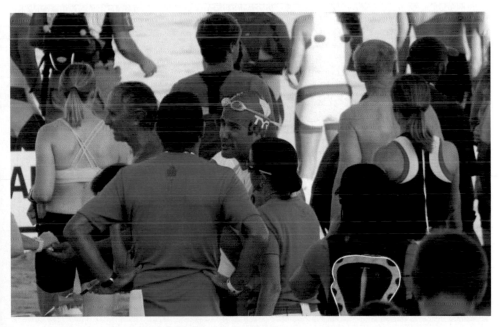

On the way to my bike, I had to ask where I could leave the glasses I needed for the swim. *Photo by Kelsey Vlieks.*

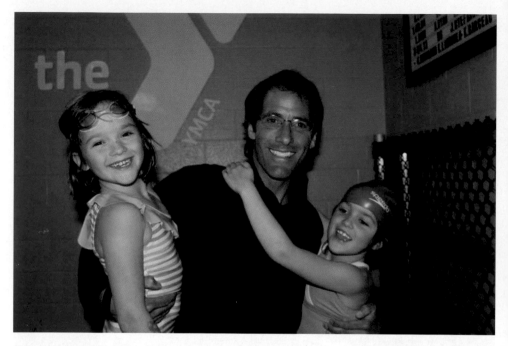

The next generation of triathletes? The girls at swim team practice at the Stonington, Connecticut, Y in August 2013. *Photo by Kelsey Vlieks.*

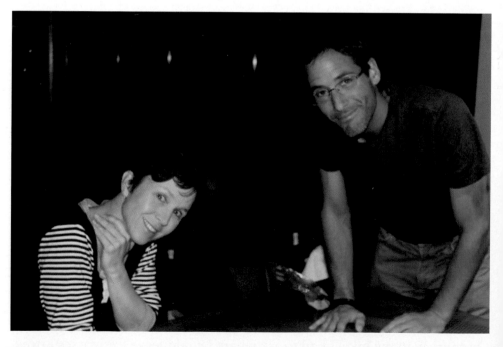

With Kelsey, visiting friends in New York City, September 2013. *Photo by Ute Vlieks.*

or nuts. After what seemed like an eternity, I reached the point where the Kentfield dietician allowed me a bit of pizza and a salad. After weeks of what tasted like bland gruel, it was astoundingly good.

Kelsey, as always, remained vigilant.

"I am starting to become a little stricter with his diet," she wrote. "It is common for head-injury patients to gain weight because their mind isn't telling them when to stop eating. That's where I come in."

I was not worried about my weight. I knew only that I was constantly hungry, and to me that was a good sign. My balance was improving, a bit anyway. I was on a slow and steady slog in the right direction.

Kelsey wrote toward the end of my Kentfield days:

"When he gets tired he still stumbles, but he's come so far from a few weeks ago. Dirk actually ran a little this week with someone holding onto him. I wish I had a video camera because it was pretty amazing, He was so happy. He seems to do better when faced with more challenging exercises, like walking on grass or running because it requires him to stay focused.

The improvement continued while we waited for the answers that would open the door to the rest of my life.

By August 17, Kelsey was able to write, "I spoke with Dirk's doctor and she mentioned that all of his therapists are thrilled with his progress. He really is wonderful. He's motivated, funny, polite, and so thankful to be here enjoying every day."

I was passing with flying colors, and we got the notice it was time to leave. I wanted to go home, and by then I was more than ready. After six steadily improving weeks, I was going home at last. I could not wait. Our second anniversary was coming up that week, and there was no better place to spend it with Kelsey than our home.

A jubilant Kelsey shared the wonderful news, as always tempered by reality:

"We will finally be back in our space together, which we are *sooo* excited about. Dirk has met his rehab goals and is now ready for home and outpatient therapies. I think he is at a point where psychologically he needs to be in his own space."

No kidding.

But while I joked and tried to divert people's attention, somewhere beneath the surface I was roiling, too. I was scared, and my cranky sleeps and stiff necks continued. While these more devious undercurrents were taking hold, I started to think about it. We have five senses. When we sleep, we lose our sense of hunger; we shut off our eyesight and close down our hearing. But we always dream, even if we are not aware of it. We can't shut down our subconscious mind. It is always at work, and mine apparently was working overtime.

As we packed and headed for home and its wonderful comfort and familiarity, we were still trying to learn what had dropped me so quickly to the ground. At Kentfield we had the benefit of being close to the prestigious University of California, San Francisco Medical Center and its unparalleled neurological unit—perhaps the country's best. As things settled and as I moved forward, away from critical care and toward the rest of my life, we began a series of tests to learn what the problem was.

It was showtime.

The first reading of the results of MRIs showed that I had a midbrain "cavernous malformation." Doctors told us it was the result of a "developmental venous anomaly." In other words, I had had a small growth in my brain that had been growing slowly all my life. It eventually had ruptured a vein.

It could have happened while I was sleeping, or watching television, or eating dinner. My exertions that day had nothing to do with anything. I could once again count my blessings it burst the vein when and where it did, so I could get immediate medical attention. It would have been all over for me if it had done so when I was out alone on a training ride, or swimming in the ocean.

At the race, the medical help was there immediately, and it saved my life.

Michael Lawton, the UCSF neurologist who explained the primary test results to Kelsey and me while we sat tensely across from him at his desk in his well-lit office, told us this malformation was like an island of blood vessels close to a prominent vein. He said it was mostly separated from the blood supply, meaning it was almost its own little entity.

Obviously, it was not too separate, because my bleeding was what they described as "massive."

He presented us with two options, neither of which was a walk in the park. There were very few surgeons in the country masterful and confident enough to take on this intricately delicate surgery. Dr. Lawton was one of them, another spot of good luck.

There are always options in surgery, usually broken down into neat statistical analyses, as if your life were a lottery. An actuarial breakdown, I suppose, is necessary. A surgeon will tell you, "If we do this type of procedure and it is successful, you have an eighty percent chance of returning to normal. But if there are complications, there's a chance you will lose your leg or you will be paralyzed or never see again."

They will lay out the pluses, then dampen them with the downsides. Numbers are unemotional—perhaps that is how a surgeon can pull himself into a state of mind to make the delicate cuts in the first place.

In my case, Dr. Lawton said I had two choices, and it depended on how much detritus had been left by the massive bleeding in the first place, much like the aftermath of an unexpected flash flood.

He told us calmly (is there ever such a thing as a nervous surgeon?) that he would try the procedure only if he could reach the malformation safely, that is, without having to cause any more damage just getting in there. We would later learn that the bleeding had indeed had created a clear path to the site, a way for the doctor to reach it—another bit of darkly tinted good luck.

But sitting in his office that Friday afternoon, none of us knew that. Kelsey and I left without knowing about that.

That made for a long weekend. How does one bide his time when waiting to learn if his chances of returning to normal hangs on something over which he has no control. The waiting is interminable; even an hour drags on as you try to control your thoughts and worries. Some people, I imagine, go worst-case scenario. We chose not to go down that path and managed to remain optimistic.

But over that long weekend, we had to mull the second option, the one we would be forced to take if Dr. Lawton could not get to the site and could not remove that malformation. That was to do nothing, and wait for what would be the next and inevitable massive bleed. The timing would again be unpredictable. It would happen, but we just would not know when. And perhaps the next time we might not be so lucky.

Statistically, I had a 10 percent chance per year another bleed would occur. That would mean it could happen again within ten years. It was inevitable, or so I thought. I'm no mathematician. The numbers game would mean that within ten years there was a chance I could possibly have another one.

I had a ticking time bomb inside my brain.

I did not want to live with that. And neither did Kelsey.

I didn't want friends looking at me askance, pretending they were not worried. I did not want to say goodnight to Kelsey and hope I'd wake up normally the next day.

"Sleep tight dear, hope I'm alive when we wake up."

That was no way to live.

The grand prize we all wanted to win was a successful surgery to remove the growth, the dark shadow that threatened the rest of my life. That was the prize as we waited.

And wait we did. We managed.

A series of appointments, each more detailed and increasingly tense as doctors zeroed in on how to proceed, lay ahead. First, Dr. Lawton and his team of neurosurgeons would study the film in minute detail to see if they wanted more defined images. We waited again while the team met to discuss the possibilities, hoping that if everything worked out, I would have the surgery.

"If we could possibly remove it, that would be incredible," Kelsey wrote to the email group—who I suppose was also waiting with tension and hope.

"Dirk and I would be able to return back to life without this anomaly hanging over our heads."

That was the hope, muted perhaps a bit by the fear.

Kelsey added a note that summed it all up.

"My head is spinning after putting all this on paper. Dirk and I are trying (and hopefully succeeding) at staying positive."

At times Kelsey would break; the emotion of it all and the strain of trying to keep it in would prove too much. The whole path ahead of us was stretched too tightly, and trying to manage with at least an edge of stoicism was futile.

"I personally have had some tough spots," Kelsey wrote, "because I have been so focused on his rehab the past four weeks and how well he is doing, that I was quickly brought back to the reality of what we are facing. It's huge and scary and it really stinks. It seems so unfair. As Dirk would say, I have had leaking eyes for a few days. We both have so much pain and sadness on the inside that I tend to cover the tear department for us."

That was the reality. I kept it on the inside, as well. But instead of crying, for me it was the torturous sleeps, my subconscious thoughts. I wonder if it would have been better if I could have just cried, just released it all in an explosive and cleansing fit of tears. But I couldn't and didn't.

And I wouldn't.

That's not how I felt. I truly don't want to go all John Wayne about it, but crying and self-pity would have been the easy way. If that was what I wanted, some self-absorbed fits of pity, I would have planted myself in a comfortable chair the first moment I got to Kentfield. I could have just sat back and watched the sunset, swilling gin-and-tonics and letting everyone else worry. I could have said, *I deserve this after all I've just been through*. I could have looked at the therapists and Kelsey and my family and friends and said, *I'm not going to do this*. And I bet no one would have objected.

But that is just not part of my nature, and I'm not sure if it is a blessing or a curse.

Instead, I worked hard and we went home. Home was so wonderful and comforting.

Kelsey announced the long-awaited move to our friends:

"There will be no more beeps and bumps in the night. Dirk will require 24-hour supervision for safety, but I am getting a wheelchair for him so he can tag along with me. Everything will take a little time, but it's worth it to have him by my side."

So we packed up our temporary and unsettled life at Kentfield and moved back to 121 Palm Avenue, our wonderful house. It had been a very long time since I closed the front door on the way to the airport for the race. It may as well have been a lifetime.

So the bittersweet mélange continued. I had done enough to go home, to truly savor the familiar smells and comforts and day-to-day memories—well enough to celebrate with the Charlie Ehm's great anniversary meal, well enough to continue my rehab exertions. But that was mixed with the fear of what would happen next.

We were home, but I was now occupying a different body under different circumstances.

"This is another adjustment that has its own set of challenges, but to have him by my side is the best," Kelsey wrote just after we settled back in.

But we were still playing a waiting game. Was I improving only to be wiped out again? It was, to say the least, an uncomfortable and exhausting thought. I suppose it was like living on a fault line after an earthquake. When is it time to give up thoughts of rebuilding and just move on, get used to the devastation and make the most of it?

We went back for several visits at UCSF. Could Dr. Lawton proceed, and would we want to? By then, we knew we were ready for the surgery, but was Dr. Lawton?

Kelsey wrote of one visit on August 17 as we neared the big decision:

"We were nervous, because it felt like so much was riding on this meeting and what he had to say. It's so hard to stay calm and composed when your nerves and emotions are all over the place. I wanted to yell or cry or both, and amazingly enough an inner strength appeared that I didn't know even existed. Where on Earth does that come from? Maybe it's that I still feel like were living in a dream (nightmare) and it will eventually end and we will wake up."

During that meeting, Dr. Lawton told us that the tests showed my malformation was relatively small—about the size of a pea. "Small" is an impotent term, though, so meaningless when we considered the devastation it had wreaked on everything and everyone. The tests also showed it was close to the surface of the brain, though there appeared to still be healthy brain tissues between the surface and the malformation.

As always, there was a caveat that would present another tough choice. The malformation was near the part of the brain that controlled my eyes—the tectum. It was possible, Dr. Lawton said, that in going in to remove the malformation, the tectum would be affected, which meant my eyes could be affected—I could lose motor control, and my eyes would roll randomly. That would affect everything from my vision to my balance. I might always see double images. I would not be able to look up and down or track movement from side to side.

I had already gone through that to a certain extent when I first woke up, but it had been steadily improving. Did I want to take the chance that the whole thing would return, and this time permanently?

One option was to wait four months for another MRI and to see if the picture would be clearer, literally and figuratively. In those four months I would continue to heal and maybe the wait would give Dr. Lawton a better idea of the risks involved.

There are always risks in surgery, especially something as delicate as brain surgery.

Going for the surgery was, to Kelsey and me, a no-brainer—and so was not waiting. We wanted the surgery, and we wanted it as soon as possible:

"I don't want us to wake up every day knowing there is a time bomb in his head. I explained to Dr. Lawton that we want to start a family and do not want to live with this hanging over us. How could I ever leave him alone? I told him we would have to get him one of those buttons to wear around his neck that automatically calls 911."

There was never really too much if any doubt about where we would opt for the surgery. Kelsey and I did everything together; that is how we had become not just a married couple, but almost a single entity.

"I think right now as a family we have decided to have the surgery," Kelsey wrote.

So we moved on and put the decision in the hands of the medical team. If they thought they could go in, we were all for it. Kelsey and I went for frequent walks. I would often think back to my first step out of bed at Kentfield. I was dizzy, nauseated from the strain. My legs buckled as I grabbed for support to take that first step, my hand on the bed. At the time, that seemed huge. Now, back home, I could walk for a half hour, and I even managed to inject short half-minute runs. To me, those first runs were like crossing the Sahara or climbing Everest, however you might want to describe it—but it was huge. I did not want to lose that progress.

So we waited for the decision. Kelsey closed her August 25 email with a heartfelt description of the situation:

"I hope these letters are helpful. It's so hard to paint an accurate picture when every day we are faced with new challenges and hardships, as well as little miracles. I was telling someone yesterday that the emotion you feel going through an experiences like this is too big to accurately describe. Part of it is tremendous sadness, but it is also happiness because he's alive. I try to stay focused on the positive and savor the moments when Dirk laughs, because laughter is the best medicine."

I felt so alive at home, and that energy allowed me to accelerate my progress. I started working on core conditioning, and more balance exercises. I made pancakes from scratch for breakfast. I went swimming, though I had somehow forgotten how to breathe while I was doing it. I felt great light and joy from doing the simplest things.

Then we heard the good news we had so badly wanted from Dr. Lawton. Further study of the MRIs showed there was a clear path to the growth, so Dr. Lawton could proceed. I put concerns about the obvious risks aside. I wanted that thing out of my head, and I wanted it out as soon as possible. I was willing to take my chances.

The intricate, computer-assisted microsurgery was expected to last six hours. Doctors would enter my brain from the back of my head, first cutting a flap of skin, then removing a portion of my skull while I sat upright. The day before, guided by previous scans, doctors had shaved patches on the back and top of my head and glued on various sensors they would use the next day to guide them. The next morning, before I was due in preop, Kelsey and I went across the street to a busy cafeteria for breakfast. With all the various wires on my bald head attached with what looked like Styrofoam earplugs, I looked like a medical experiment gone bad—some sort of renegade automaton. I enjoyed watching the reactions of the diners, who could not seem to avoid staring. I don't blame them for wondering. I guess it says something about my state of mind that I was hungry. I was not nervous and went right for my favorite—a big stack of comforting pancakes.

Shortly before surgery, doctors took one more MRI. It showed there was still a lot of blood remaining from the initial burst. That would make things a bit dicier, but Dr. Lawton was confident he could proceed. Before we went to the operating room, he asked me once more if I wanted to wait, if I wanted more time to see if things would clear.

I asked him if waiting would make a difference to him, if he would do anything different with more information.

"Probably not," he said.

"Then let's get it done," I told him.

And so he did. The successful procedure lasted five hours and was clean in every way. Dr. Lawton did not have to intrude anywhere near my tectum, so my eye control was unaffected.

My enemy was gone, finite, disappeared into a laboratory jar for a test of its pathology—the last and final straw in the process. Good riddance.

The next morning, while I was still groggy from nearly half a day of surgery, Dr. Lawton brought Kelsey and me in to review the scans. My malformation, he told us, was more akin to a slow-growing tumor, and I had likely had it since I was born. It had reached the point where it had grown enough to intrude on a nearby blood vessel and burst it.

Buoyed by the results, exhausted but comforted the long wait was over, my head looking like a roadmap; but even as we knew the malicious growth was gone, another wait began.

Was this tumor malignant? It was a short wait, and I think in a way we were too tired and relieved to worry. No, it was not, the pathology results revealed the next day.

The morning I went in for surgery, there were two other patients scheduled for the same procedure. I was first. There was a man set to go in after me who had a similar growth that had only recently been discovered. He had had no symptoms until several unusual headaches had prompted him to get an MRI. He had until only a week before lived a normal life. It turned out his tumor was malignant.

I thought about that. My circumstances were far different. Unlike that man, I had had ample warning that something was wrong. I was laid low, crippled in fact, and had spent almost three months working myself back. I still had a long road ahead of me—but it was a road that was now filled with hope.

That poor man likely did not know what had hit him, and he was certainly facing a much darker future with a malignant tumor.

I was the lucky one.

Eight

TO THE TOP OF MOUNT TAM

I was not aware I was missing something in my life. I was too busy to sit back and do an audit on the various things I was doing. I was not inclined to be introspective anyway. I didn't have the luxury or inclination toward self-analysis. Everything I was doing before I met Kelsey was full and rewarding, and with my training friends and the various orbits we traveled, things were interesting and energizing. It was all good. Throw in work, which I enjoyed as much as anyone can enjoy work, and I was a very contented guy.

I'm sure it is not only me, but sometimes—most times, really—people are not aware something is missing until it arrives, usually unannounced. Once this unexpected gift shows, two things happen. They look back and wonder, stupefied at how they had somehow managed to survive. They wonder how they even managed. Then they look ahead and realize their life will never be the same.

I'm not sure what it was for me. Was it fear of change? Inertia? Being a bonehead? I don't know, and it really doesn't matter. The empirical and undisputed truth is that once I met Kelsey Zeigler, my life was never the same again.

I was not even looking, to tell the truth. Things were calm and moving in the right direction—wherever that was. I was happy with that. I certainly wasn't lonely or lovelorn or anything close to it. I was just contentedly bobbing in the current, not really minding which way it was taking me.

Kelsey hit me like a tsunami.

In fact, I was so unconcerned about my social life, I had to be dragged out the night I met Kelsey. At the time, I had not thought too far beyond what occupied my days. Work was fulfilling, in the odd way that work can be when you don't hate your job. The rest was simple, too. I worked out, which I loved. I went out with friends, mostly hanging out my training partners, since we were basically in the same orbit. I raced. I wasn't in love, and I was not desperate to be involved with someone. Everything I was doing meshed in a neat, organized, dedicated, and well-oiled life.

Meeting Kelsey changed everything, in the electrifying way that only falling in love can change your life. I did not stop what I was doing. I didn't quit my job, or give up working out or start writing poetry or leave my friends for another life. Kelsey and I joined each other the first moment we met. It was as simple as that—a wonderful karmic chemistry that united us instantly and has kept us tied to each other ever since.

Kelsey and I met at a benefit, both dragged there by friends. It took one dance for me to know I wanted to marry her.

As soon as Kelsey and I spoke on the dance floor, the crazy idea was cemented, at least in my mind. I even told friends my plans before Kelsey had made it back to her table after the dance. After that, there were a few minor things I had to take care of, like getting her phone number and trying to gauge if the feeling was mutual. But I managed.

At the time, I was doing computer work for iBeam Broadcasting in suburban Sunnyvale. It was work I enjoyed that came with a good paycheck. iBeam was at the time involved in developing ways to stream audio and video to Internet users, so it was a cutting-edge sort of thing. But cutting edge means risk, I guess. I was blissfully unaware the company was going broke. It eventually filed for Chapter 11 bankruptcy. It didn't really matter to me one way or the other, though. It was work. I enjoyed a nice paycheck that allowed me to live downtown and do my triathlon things, which by then had totally absorbed me.

Kelsey was working for the Celebration Fantastic, a company that offered knickknacks, gifts, and collectibles that it called "wonderful witty whatnots."

We were both enjoying our lives, and neither of us was looking for a partner. We certainly weren't heavy into the dating scene. Kelsey had her friends, and I had my circle of workout partners and training friends whose company I relished.

Kelsey was enjoying the energy of the city, and I was contented with my busy schedule. Between working out and work, I didn't have a lot of time to ponder the meaning of life or lament lost loves.

I had vowed to myself that I would not get involved with a triathlete. Needless to say, there were plenty of attractive and supremely fit and fun women in the groups I hung around with. But it didn't seem like a good idea to me to mix romance with training —strange as that might sound. My self-imposed restriction might seem contrary to the usual rules of dating, but it worked out well for me.

Kelsey was an athlete. She had played rugby, softball, and squash in college and was an enthusiastic runner. She just was not as obsessed with triathlon as I had become.

It was a triathlon event that brought us together for that first life-changing hello. Two of my friends had cajoled me into attending a dinner-dance and fashion show to benefit Team In Training, which raised money for The Leukemia & Lymphoma Society.

"Sure," I said. "Why not?"

Meanwhile, Kelsey had gone through the same reluctant concession. "Why not?" she said to her friend, Jody Young, who as it turned out was also a friend of mine.

The gears were beginning to mesh.

At the benefit, I was sitting at a table talking, enjoying the sounds of soothing and rhythmic Brazilian jazz—the sort of music you can't help but get pulled into. I had lived in Brazil, after all.

I saw Kelsey coming across the room, right toward me.

She asked if I wanted to dance. What happened next is still a matter of debate. I thought I had danced exceptionally well. Kelsey thought I had two left feet. It doesn't matter. Before we even finished the dance, I was totally in over my head. In the blink of an eye I was toast, mesmerized.

After the dance we smiled and headed back to our own tables. As I sat down, I announced that I would marry that girl who had just danced with me. They smiled but said nothing.

A few days later I ran into a friend who had been sitting with Kelsey, and I asked if she thought Kelsey would mind if I called her. She told me it would be fine. Kelsey had mentioned me, she said. The wheels were in motion, the deck was stacked.

I called Kelsey the next week and asked her out.

I guess it would not seem unusual to note that our first date was a trail run up the stunning Mount Tam—Mount Tamalpais —a Mecca for runners in Marin County. Right across the Golden Gate bridge, Mount Tam is laced with challenging trails starting right at the bottom from Stinson Beach to its top—Troop 80, Bootjack, Matt Davis, dozens of other places to run and soak it all in. At many points on the way up, you can stop and turn to see jaw-dropping views of San Francisco Bay, the bridge, and San Francisco itself. Mount Tam is a magnet for runners. Why wouldn't it be? I love Mount Tam. There are more than 300 miles of winding trails, most of them leading at some point to its crest and the view of the bay 2,500 feet below. If the weather is clear and the wind in the right direction, you can even catch a glimpse of the snow-covered Sierra Madre, one hundred fifty miles away.

It turned out that Kelsey had been working out with Team In Training, a triathlon group, but was not as hard core as I had become. By the time we were fifty yards into our run, like a skillful lawyer, I had deleted my self-imposed "no triathlete" clause. I never gave it another thought again. Funny how those things work out.

After our run, around one o'clock on a stunning bright afternoon, we drove over to the Cactus Café in Mill Valley, a great Mexican place. We started talking. We kept talking. The conversation flowed from one thing to another, swirling around laughs and old stories and clear, short flashes of who we were and where we wanted to go. We talked of the usual things—our backgrounds, our friends, our lives. Time passed quickly, though I would not have known. I noticed only Kelsey smiling and effortless, talking across from me at the table. I did not notice anything else. That is, until the manager came over and politely told us they were closing. We had spent the entire afternoon caught up in each other.

I drove Kelsey back into the city to her apartment in the Marina District. We talked for two more hours, sitting in my car outside.

What did we find so interesting to talk so intently about for so long? I have no idea, really. The conversation just flowed so naturally, effortlessly.

And so it began.

Time doesn't really enforce itself on you when you're totally wrapped up in someone. But it was not long before Kelsey was spending more time at my place than hers. She kept her apartment, but, in reality, she had moved in with me.

There were no secrets between us, including the unimpeachable fact that we would marry. That was a given end result of the mysterious chemistry that had brought us together. I knew I wanted to propose, and Kelsey knew I wanted to propose. But for some reason something always intervened and I couldn't seem to pull the trigger.

So we settled into a different type of dance from the seductive samba that started the whole thing. I waited for the right time; Kelsey waited for me to do it. I wasn't happening, though, and I think at some point Kelsey just threw it to the winds, adopting more of an "it will happen when it happens" kind of perspective. Kelsey has always been an unflinching pragmatist. She was a Zen master.

Kelsey's stoicism was the perfect antidote for my own ineptness.

I had a plan, though. More than anything, I wanted to surprise her. By then, we were spending pretty much all our time together, so it was an ambitious plan.

One afternoon, I planned to ask the big question on the steps leading up to Point Reyes lighthouse, with its breathtaking views of the Pacific in the distance. When we reached the spot, I realized I had forgotten the ring.

I knew I needed to focus, and quickly.

I came up with another plan.

I had been training for the Mount Tam Hill Climb, a popular race that attracted hundreds of runners. It was as close to a celebration of running as anything. I had always enjoyed the vibes of that upbeat race, a music-filled family kind of event.

It was a grueling race, up stairs and along narrow sagebrush-lined trails and through sweet pine-scented groves where watching your footing was as important as pace and endurance. One Sunday, after I'd done my usual long Sunday workout, I was sitting at the dining room table reading the *Chronicle* and wolfing down my usual burrito when I casually asked Kelsey if she wanted to head out to Mount Tam so I could check out the route I planned for the race. I posed it as an innocent, spontaneous question, but I had put a lot of work into planning the rest of the afternoon.

"Want to go?" I asked.

"Not really," she said.

My best-laid plans began to unravel seconds after Kelsey's disinterested reply.

"C'mon. It's a brilliant day today. Just come along. It'll be a great afternoon and you'll be outside."

"Sure, why not?" she replied, not exactly jumping to the door.

I was of course relieved, because I had planned the rest of the afternoon with the intricacy of the D-Day invasion.

I had packed a bottle of champagne and two fluted glasses. And this time, I remembered the ring.

I had made dinner reservations at El Paseo, an upscale restaurant in Mill Valley for later that evening. I had stashed more formal clothes for both of us in the trunk of my Subaru.

I dragged the wavering Kelsey to the car.

To get into the park, we had to slide under a gate rail that closed off the entrance to cars. Kelsey knelt and scampered under the thick wooden rail but stood too soon and banged her back against its sharp edge. Already less than enthused about heading up the trail, she swore and stood slowly.

I looked at her expectantly, worried she was about to head back to the car.

I said nothing and waited.

She stretched and started walking up the trail.

I had dodged the bullet.

We hiked casually and steadily to the crest, a hike of about an hour. The soft breezes and steady sunshine through the trees hitting the path were a perfect antidote for Kelsey's mood. I knew it would be. Innately optimistic and effervescent, Kelsey was incapable of holding a bad mood for any length of time.

We reached the crest and stood looking down at the Bay and the bridge and the city in the distance. It was a vista we never tired of.

I reached into my backpack quickly, calmly, and brought out the ring and held it in my clasped palms.

I proposed.

Kelsey just stared at me and the ring, dumbstruck, stunned that I had finally done what we both had known I would do for months.

She kept staring but said nothing.
She smiled broadly, excitedly, beamingly.
It was a stunning, frozen moment.
It was nothing short of perfect, that moment.
Kelsey is the love of my life, and the life of my love.

Nine

THE GIFT OF ORDINARY

The jagged emotional arc that began the moment I swung off my bike in a daze on the Queen K to the recovery room at UCSF had always been electrified with fear. There were no lulls and few moments of serenity. Each day began with the same question: Would I be alive this time tomorrow? The question was there in the ICU at Queen's, it hovered unsaid at Kentfield as I began to wake up, and it blared while we waited for the biopsy results.

Living in that taut world for three months will give you a different perspective on life. It transforms every breath and sign of progress into bright and welcome light. Fighting to stay on the right side of the equation tends to make the simplest things stunning and the difficult ones miraculous.

Every day was about life or death. Summoning the energy to win more time kept me looking forward to the next sunrise. I knew I would give as much as I could to beat this thing.

There was immense relief after the tumor was removed and we learned it was benign, of course. And gratitude for everyone whose support and love had helped pull me through. But after that welcome news, the pulsing, almost continuous energy injected by the fear of whether I would even live was replaced by a much bigger challenge—the banality of what lay ahead.

There is not a lot of drama in constant repetition with no end in sight. It can be suffocating if you let it be. There is very little excitement in daily therapy routines that rarely produce noticeable signs of improvement. The work ahead for me would bring minuscule notches of good news only after months of work.

At first, before the real work began, Kelsey let everyone know the stunning results. On September 12, she wrote: "Dirk's surgery could not have gone better. The surgeon did not have to cut through the tectum, so Dirk's eyes look great. He is having minimal left-sided weakness and he says his butt hurts like the Dickens (that's because he was in a seated position)."

She added something that would prove omniscient, though at the time it was more of a lilting chirpiness, a sign of hope.

"Oh Boy, I am glad we are through with this! It was a very challenging day, but as with everything these days, there are lessons to be learned and strength to be gained. And now Dirk and I can continue to rehab, rehab, rehab until he is back where he wants to be."

By September 18, I was home when Kelsey wrote her next note to our friends. In it she recounted the transition. The lengthy surgery and four days in bed without moving had put a hit on the progress I had been making. Before the operation I was walking almost forty-five minutes without having to stop and rest. At home at first, I could manage only twenty minutes.

She briefly recounted her own relief: "I can't express how wonderful it is to be through this surgery and have him home for good. Prior to surgery it was hard for me to feel real happiness because there was always an underlying angst. But it's getting easier to laugh and not have such a heavy heart. I feel there is a lightness in my step that I have not felt since June 3. I no longer wake up at 3 a.m. and have to talk myself out of not worrying—ninety-five percent of the worrying is gone. I realize we still have a long road of recovery in front of us, months and months, but he's going to be OK."

I was feeling something quite different.

As I sat on the front porch of our house on Palm Avenue, awash in the comfort of familiar things that had been missing for months, the immensity of what had happened began to sink in. What lay ahead did not involve high-explosive drama or fireworks. I knew what lay ahead were, long, repetitive, achingly boring rehab workouts that would show only painstakingly slow progress. Tedium.

And with that reality came another revelation. I did not have a condition that would at some point clear up. What gradually sunk in was the cold fact that I was not afflicted with a disease from which I would eventually be cured. There was only debris—and it was up it me to clear up the mess as well as I could.

I would live, I realized. But the bigger question was how would I live? What would my life be like now that I had survived? I won the first phase. I would have a life. But as I sat in those early days on my front porch, my cat Mouse purring contentedly on my lap as I watched traffic roll by, I wondered.

Life, yes. But what kind of life?

Before the event I once could run hard, train hard, eat well, and see straight. I lived joyously and energetically. While sitting on the porch, I took an assessment. I could not see straight. I had very little balance, my speech was unclear, my facial expressions seemingly disconnected. I could see straight only with glasses. The things that had driven me and motivated me, that had marked me as the person I once was were now all gone.

In many ways, the only time I would appear normal was outside a bar at closing time, when the drunks reeled out the door.

I am not inclined to self-pity and never was. Self-pity is a tumor more lethal and destructive than the one that had laid me out. I have no time for that. But a brief flash of self-pity nearly pulled me in and brought me down.

Almost.

One afternoon, walking unsteadily home after yet another therapy session at Kentfield, I paused on a pedestrian bridge over a small canal cross Magnolia Avenue and watched the traffic passing by unaffectedly and steadily at fifty miles an hour. I had been fighting to keep my balance the whole way home. I couldn't see straight. I was tired from too many sleepless nights and bad dreams. I was down, at the lowest point in my life.

The whole situation—the event, the drama, the damage, the intensive care and the surgery, the whole mess, simply did not seem real. But it was real, and there was nothing I could do to change a thing.

The thought, nothing more than a flash, really, came quickly. I could very easily just step quickly off the side of the road and drop into the path of one of the cars. The driver would have no time to react, and it would be over quickly—for me anyway. The others—Kelsey, my parents, her parents, our friends—would mourn, but then they could move on. They would be free of the whole mess. I was holding people down instead of letting them blossom.

There was nothing planned about that black thought. I had not sat morosely devising my demise. It just appeared, uncontrolled, spontaneous, and unbidden.

At the moment, that instant, I had to summon everything that was right and good about my life. And I did.

The dark moment passed as quickly as the car that would have sent me flying. Morose, self-defeating thoughts were not my strong suit. If they were, I would have never made it out of the intensive care unit at Queen's.

I walked the rest of the way home and said nothing. The entire bizarre urge frightened me more than anything I had experienced.

It would be a year before I would mention it to Kelsey, that frightening, paralyzing instant of self-pity that had so briefly overwhelmed me.

That frightening moment would lock in a resolve that has served me well ever since. I stepped back from the edge of the road and knew that I would be fine with whatever lay ahead. I had beaten the odds. I was alive and moving. I would simply keep moving—but in the right direction.

Bob Seger once wrote a great lyric: "I wish I didn't know now what I didn't know then." It is a stunning line for a number of reasons, not the least of which is its compressed power—an entire biography in eleven words.

When I got home that afternoon, I went right to the sun on the front porch and sat and watched that steady traffic from an entirely new perspective. I took a deep breath as the cat crawled onto my lap. I soaked up the life of it—that stunningly normal scene that seemed so far beyond my reach twenty minutes before.

I would focus. I would not look back. I would move ahead one dull tedious painfully boring step ahead at time. And I would improve every single day. I was good. I was alive. I would get better.

Ten

UPWARD, SLOWLY

As I look back on it now ten years later I can see the roots of what had worn me down and so suddenly assaulted me on that bridge over Magnolia Avenue. It had begun with frightening dreams I started recalling during the sleepless nights at Kentfield, but it accelerated in the recovery room at UCSF.

I slowly woke up after close to five hours of surgery, my grogginess penetrated by the sharp, piercing screams of another patient. She was begging for something—anything—to deaden her pain, actually yelling, "Please help me." Nurses were asking the doctors if anything could be done.

The doctors were saying no. She has reached her limit of drugs, they said. We can do nothing more. The nurses were frustrated, the doctors unmoved. The woman continued to moan.

Welcome back to the real world.

I had my own wake-up disturbances, as well. For the delicate surgery, my head had been taped firmly to the chair in which I had reclined while surgeons went into my brain behind me. A band of tape ran across my lower lip, anchoring my head. As I awoke, the tape and its resoluteness in keeping me from moving began to annoy me while I was still half under. Without consciously trying to do so, I began to chew it off, and with it came part of my lower lip, skin mostly. It was a little grisly reminder of where I was and what had happened. And later, of course, it hurt like hell.

While I was still in the recovery room, I began absentmindedly scratching my ear, picking out what felt like tiny bits of abrasive sand. Odd, I thought. What I had been trying to remove was actually gruesome sawdust of a different sort—tiny bits of bone from the surgeons cutting open the back of my skull that nurses had forgotten to clean out.

By the time I was in the recovery room at UCSF, I had not had a good night's sleep in weeks. The dreams I began having at Queen's were starting to come back to me, frightening and disturbing. By the time I was at Kentfield, getting any kind of restful comforting sleep had become a major effort. Sleeping on either side was not possible. I tried but just could not manage it. So I would sleep on my back, which I had never done, and which I found both uncomfortable and annoying. Naturally, once I fell asleep I would roll to one side or the other, then wake with a start and try my back again.

After the surgery, sleeping on my back was not an option, either. One early night after the surgery, my head seemed to snag on the pillow, caught by a jagged bone fragment on the incision that had not yet meshed. I reached back and pulled it out.

Any extended hospital stay is rarely smooth, and my own time at Queen's, at Kentfield, and at UCSF was not without its own irritation, if not peril. Doctors had nicked my femoral artery putting in a shunt, and I nearly bled to death. A nurse had mistakenly given me a pill instead of a liquid dose of medication, and I nearly choked. Another nurse calmly dripped hydrogen peroxide into my eyes, not noticing she was using the wrong bedside vial, which was jolting and very painful—if not dangerous.

It was not any single one of these things that had beaten me down, but rather an accumulation—a barrage of small irritations whose sum total ended up being more than I could manage, I guess.

Maybe that's what did it.

Or was it something else that began to sink in as I looked at what lay ahead? The life I had known was not coming back after a few therapy sessions and the right medicine. It was a dangerous sort of introspection, the kind of analysis that can take you down the wrong road. I ventured a few steps in that dark direction. That was what hit me on the bridge that day, I'm afraid. I'm sure it was a natural reaction, but it was powerful and frightening nonetheless. I was exhausted and for that instant could not imagine what lay ahead or summon the energy to fight it. It was a spontaneous surrender, an almost overwhelming urge to lift my hand to the sky and give the finger to the cosmos.

Whatever it was, it was over in a flash.

That's not to say we were marching to a dirge the entire time at UCSF. The fact that the insidious tumor was gone was nothing short of wonderful. Even better was the fact that it was not malignant. We would have another scare about a growth at the site later, but for the moment we were home free and could not have been happier about it.

There were lighter moments, and Kelsey and I were always able to find them—and appreciate them. Laughter can cure almost anything, and we did laugh.

Kelsey made the mistake of getting a small slice of pepperoni pizza for herself at the hospital cafeteria. After days of bland, soft, and tasteless hospital food I wanted that pizza. I begged Kelsey to let me have a bite. I was unrelenting and I wore her down, which I knew I could do, despite her usual fastidiousness about diet.

She cut it in half and passed it across the table. As I was jamming it down, I coughed a bit. Nothing serious, mind you, no more than a result of me cramming it into my mouth and forgetting to chew. Kelsey bolted upright, ran behind me, and started a Heimlich, much to the amazement of everyone else sitting around us. As soon as I could swallow, I smiled and told her she could sit back down, I was fine.

Later, leaving the hospital with Kelsey pushing my wheelchair at speed, the wheels locked up solid. Everything stopped but me. I was barely able to catch myself from doing a header onto the concrete ramp. That would have prompted an ironic return to the emergency room—a guy who had just had brain surgery coming back in before he had even left. We laughed on the way home.

Home. Yes, that was a sweet moment.

I was so incredibly happy to be home. One of our first visitors was Kiki Silver, who removed my stitches. Then we settled in among everything that was so comforting—the aromas, the cats, the lighting, the familiar, anything that did not look like the inside of a hospital room.

That initial burst of euphoria would slowly begin to deflate and lead to that moment on the bridge. After I stepped from the edge of the road that day, I resolved almost instantly to do whatever I needed to do to get back to where I had been. But it was a tough adjustment at first.

"Look back at the past, just don't stare," a visiting friend had told me at one point early on, when I was caught briefly in a lament about the past four months and the unfairness it all. He was trying to tell me to get what I could from what happened, maybe even mourn a bit. But don't live in it, don't dwell on it. What's done is done.

Even Kelsey had noticed my moments. In an early letter she had written, "all in all we are doing okay."

"We had a few tough days this week," she continued. "In some ways the past four months have seemed like a lifetime, but in reality we are only beginning this journey, Thank goodness Dirk is no longer in critical care, but our life has still taken a huge blow and we are trying to adjust. I think my brain is starting to come out of the initial shock and starting to face reality."

Kelsey did not know about my moment on the bridge, but she did notice I was trying to do some adjusting myself, and I was having problems with it.

"Dirk is becoming more and more aware of his deficits; he feels trapped in a slow body."

I did indeed feel trapped. But Kelsey noticed something else, and that was after my epiphany that I was in it for the long haul.

"Dirk said after an emotional conversation, 'Every day is a gift.' Isn't that the truth? For us, this fight for our life together has just begun."

After some time at home to simply let this percolate and settle, I began what Kelsey and I would later call our buckshot approach to therapy. If something offered even a glimmer of hope, we did it.

Work, repeat. Work again. I exchanged my fear of boredom and my natural inclination to want immediate and discernible results with a resolve to slowly erode the barriers that lay ahead. I would simply and forcefully put my head down knock them off, one step at a time.

I turned the mundanity of balance exercises or speech therapy or short wobbly runs into a game. Each numbing exercise, each meditation session, each drill would bring me one step closer to my old self. A completed day was a paycheck, money in the bank—whatever you want to call it. That was the prize. I decided I would take a blue-collar approach to the whole thing, like the guys on an auto assembly line. Punch in, work, punch out. Don't whine. Get the check.

I had to remind myself in those moments of self-pity that most people who had the type of stroke that knocked me down did not survive. And if they did, they did not survive well.

I would do both.

One of the first things I did was to attend to my almost constant double vision. Not seeing clearly affected just about everything I tried to do. I would have very brief moments of being able to see straight, often at night. But by morning everything would double up again. For that we would try acupuncture and special glasses.

Then we were off and running.

Kelsey assembled a great team and organized an ambitious effort to put the hammer down, noting in one of her earlier letters that "We have a wonderful team of therapists helping him work on his voice, gait, strength, computer skills and his cooking."

We joined the Marin Brain Injury Network and began attending weekly classes that were designed to support and encourage people with injuries like mine. There is comfort in numbers and solidarity in knowing you are not alone.

Later we would meet Bob and Lee Woodruff. Bob, a popular anchor and reporter for ABC News, was severely injured in Iraq in 2006 when a roadside bomb exploded, nearly killing him. He spent thirty-six days in a medically induced coma. Kelsey wrote to our friends of the comfort meeting Lee Woodruff and sharing the burdens:

"It was really special for me to meet a woman who understands what I've been through. Riding the elevator up to the ICU and not knowing what the day had in store, treasuring the small miracles, and dealing with the punches. It felt like a boxing ring sometimes. What else could they throw at us? Pneumonia, DVT, UTI, hydrocephalus, respiratory distress, and a second bleed?"

I had acupuncture treatments, eye therapy, balance work. I tried an antigravity treadmill. Kelsey put me on a new diet to increase blood flow, sleep therapy, speech therapy, massage, mysterious Eastern medicine, brain therapy, and meditation.

I was game, though I have to admit it was more of a "let's throw this against the wall and see if it sticks" approach.

I began serious physical therapy under the supervision of my friends Paul Lundgren and Chris Chorak, who graciously made their Presidio Sport & Medicine facilities on Gorgas Drive in Mill Valley available to me to me anytime I wanted.

Paul took me for my first swim, which proved disastrous. Before that afternoon reentry into the pool, swimming was something I had loved and had been good at. I could knock off a 100-yard freestyle in under a minute fairly easily. Swimming had been a triathlon strong suit. But as I stood on the edge of the pool that afternoon, I realized I was afraid. The thought of getting back into the water was overwhelming. I slid in and pushed off.

I had forgotten everything. I could not stroke properly. I could not stay on a straight course without Paul's guidance. More frightening, I could not breathe and ended up swallowing what felt like most of the pool. It was not a confidence builder, to say the least.

Like many other simple things that had come so naturally to me—to most people, actually—I was starting all over again, like a young child in the beginner's swimming program at the local Y.

More jarring was that I was overwhelmed with a fear of the water. My loss of control over everything that had come so naturally scared the hell out of me. I began wearing a flotation belt just to get into the water.

Later, I would use that belt for stability to run in place in the water, something I would do as often as I could. It was a safe and good workout. No falling, steady resistance, good mileage. It was boring beyond belief. I could do it for hours, though. Friends who would volunteer so graciously to keep me company while I plodded away in the shallow end, going nowhere slowly, would rarely last more than fifteen minutes. I could not blame them.

But the thing is, I swam. Every day I fought those fears and every day I got back in the water. Within two weeks I could make 100 yards without interruption. It took twenty minutes, but I could do it. That was called progress.

By then, the reality that everything would be different had sunk in: learning to speak clearly; Kelsey's choking phobia aside, learning to swallow; learning to walk without reeling and then to run; learning to control my facial muscles and basic things like picking up a cup of coffee without spilling. I was a child again, learning everything from square one.

Nothing would come quickly, though I did absorb one lesson fairly soon into the process. It was a valuable lesson in something that had never been a strong suit: patience.

This thing would require a vast reservoir of patience, I knew. So be it.

And with my newfound patience, or at least a glimmer of it, I had brain sessions in which the therapist worked with me to control my breathing, which would in turn lower my pulse rate. The therapist would use strobe lights that she professed would pick up energy and move it around, presumably to the right places.

I did vision therapy. In one drill we did often, an ophthalmologist from UCSF would hold the end of a two-foot string on the tip of my nose and slowly move the far end in her other hand from one side to the other, or up and down, and ask me to follow it with my eyes.

I locked into a simple mantra. I would do whatever was asked, and I would move forward and make everything better, even if signs of progress were barely noticeable. I conceded there was no magic bullet out there, no instant cure that would make the whole nightmare disappear. It would be a matter of degrees. It would be fine.

I would work for it, and that was no different from what I had always done.

As June 3 approached, an anniversary neither of us wanted to celebrate, I simply put it out of my mind. It would be another day. I was not going to stare at it. I was not going to dwell on it or wring my hands or somehow mark the ignominy of what happened. That would be too simple, too predictable.

I woke up, I went to rehab, I did speech therapy and physical therapy.

The day came and went.

Kelsey had a harder time with it, of course, but she had borne the burdens and the strain more than I. For Kelsey, that first anniversary was a tough one.

We moved on, slowly forward.

Eleven

ALOHA

As the anniversary approached, Kelsey would at times turn to me and tell me how terrible that day had been. She would say how utterly frightening it was to recognize my bare legs jutting from the gurney in the medical tent while doctors hovered over me frantically trying to get some sort of response. Only a few minutes before, she had been soaking up the sun and texting friends to find out where I was. A slightly disruptive fear that I might have had a flat tire and dropped out was replaced very quickly with something more grippingly ominous.

The hierarchy of what was important in life had collapsed in that one instant in the tent.

Kelsey wanted to go back to Hawaii. I was ambivalent. I was bothered mostly by my first "Did Not Finish" and had spent the better part of the year doing everything I could to get back to the point where I would finish. At that point, a year later, I was still working on walking normally. I just wasn't sure if I wanted to go back so soon.

As usual, Kelsey won the debate.

Kelsey needed to replace that frightening, adhesive memory. She had not been able to shake it off for the entire year. We talked about it as the anniversary approached and my own recovery was moving forward. I am an impatient man, and I was not where I wanted to be. Being alive was nice, I had to admit. But I still had a very long way to go. I was not sure I wanted to announce that to the world, and I was not sure I wanted to stare at it so soon.

Still, I had had a pretty good year as I looked back on it.

In Kelsey's view, we needed to banish those horrific memories with something far more palatable—something else she could lock into and smile about. We needed to spend the anniversary of the day when everything changed doing something more pleasant than hanging out in emergency tents and ambulances and life flights to Queen's.

We would return to Hawaii, and we would finish the day that had taunted us for the past year with a nice dinner and gentleness and hope. We'd meet it head-on, confront it, then we'd banish that day from our lives.

For Kelsey, the return would be cleansing and palliative. For me, the trip would be a bit more complicated.

We left San Francisco as we had the year before, on a plane for Honolulu that would get us to the Big Island, Hawaii, in time for the Honu Half Ironman, the race that did me in. This time of course, I didn't have to worry about packing the bike or anything else I had needed to race the year before.

Going back would give me the chance to close out a day that had been incomplete to me for a year. I remembered nothing of it from the moment I pulled off the bike. I would be able to somehow reconnect the dots, to try to calmly restore some vague sense of order on the accelerated entropy that had governed my life ever since that moment.

On the mainland, where psychological epiphanies at the time were more likely to be imparted on television by Oprah and Dr. Phil, I think what both Kelsey and I were looking for would have been called *closure*. We would return to the scene, see the athletes and the highway and the tents and the excitement and the hospital. We would retrace our steps, and that would somehow help. That was the general thought, anyway.

I am not a big fan of the word or concept of *closure*—as if you can simply hermetically seal off a horrific memory and never think of it again. It is a tough concept to swallow when every uneasy step you take reminds you of that day. You can't just close it off and forget it when it is in your face every waking moment.

But you can find a way to use it to propel you forward.

What we found in the islands on that first anniversary visit was not closure but something more akin to the concept of *aloha*. For people fortunate enough to live in Hawaii, *aloha* is more than a word that can be used as either hello or good-bye. It is used to express love; it is a way of life. Grasping the concept of *aloha* means you have everything you need to blend with the natural world. It is sometimes called "The Aloha Spirit," an attitude more than a simple word. It means gentleness and acceptance. It goes beyond any definition you can find about it in the dictionaries. In Hawaii, you hear *aloha* all the time and you are treated with *aloha* everywhere.

In Hawaii, we said good-bye to the demons and hello to the rest of our lives. That was much nicer than closure.

Kelsey put the whole struggle into perspective in her first note in July to friends after we returned from that cleansing trip back:

"We made it through June. Sorry I have not written sooner, but I needed to get through last month. There were a handful of days when I would turn to Dirk and tell him how awful that day was last summer."

Now that it was over, she wrote how she and I could move ahead in my recovery:

"Our trip to Hawaii was very special. We had goals in mind before we set off on our journey—let's replace the bad memories with the good and let's try to relax and enjoy ourselves in a place that Dirk had always loved. All in all, we were pretty successful in accomplishing our goals with the help of our friends in Hawaii."

Sitting briefly on my couch in my usual place in the sun on our front porch, I was able to digest the last year shortly after we returned. The first anniversary had come and gone, and I hoped there would be many more, each becoming less frantic until they faded away completely. It would be nice, I thought, to have the day pass and not even remember it.

The past year had been more than a catalog of daily rehab sessions and training and therapies. It had been a pretty good year.

I thought about something I had read during one of the rare chances I had to take a break. It was a more elegant take on Nike's "no pain, no gain." It was a quote from French playwright Pierre Corneille I had come across by accident on the Internet.

To tell the truth, I don't know much about him other that he was considered one of the great seventeenth-century dramatists. He most likely was not writing about triathlons, but he did seem to know about struggle and its benefits.

I liked the quote: "To win without risk is to triumph without glory."

I had done a lot of risking in the past year. I had taken some chances, pushed it a bit. I had started running, conquered my new fear of the water, and gotten back on the bike. I annoyed the doctors to the point where they told me that I could now work out with more vigor. When I had first started pushing it, everyone was afraid it could bring on another incident. That had been the elephant in the room, and I could see it in everyone's eyes. The thing was, I was not worried about it. I was ready to exert myself.

I had already thought of it, and the Hawaii trip only reinforced the idea. At some point I would go back and I would finish that Hona bike ride.

For me, our anniversary trip back to Hawaii was bittersweet. We accomplished Kelsey's goal of replacing the bad memories with better ones, but it was at times difficult to swallow what had happened. Going back to the race a year later was very tough for me, though. I was a spectator, not a competitor. I watched the people prep for the race, and I felt my adrenaline start pumping. This time there would be no frantic elbow-flying jostle at the start of the swim, or a long, windblown ride, or a testing run. There would be no satisfying finish.

I was instead treated to a spectator's view of something I had done with such joy before. We did get to see many old friends, quite a few of whom had been getting Kelsey's emails and who had followed my progress throughout the year. Being there, being with them, soaking up the vibes of the race and the whole scene was in a way restorative—kindling on the fire, so to speak. But it was not the real thing. I was an outsider.

But I took solace from that, and I would use it. I knew by that time it was better to embrace the realty than to live in the past. That group of friends and fellow athletes was extremely helpful while we were on the Big Island.

Tougher than watching the start was driving out to "the spot"—the geographic center that indelibly marked the onset of my new life. We pulled the car off the Queen K and parked near the sign that read Hawaii City Limits. As a token of remembrance, and to perhaps appease the fates that had so indelicately given us a year from Hell, I knelt and put a bouquet of sweet and colorful blue ginger, bougainvillea, and evening primrose at the base of the signpost.

Kelsey watched silently behind me. I stood and we looked at each other, then reached out and lightly touched the sign.

Aloha. Hello. Good-bye.

I could not say a thing for a minute or two. Kelsey chose not to, either.

Kelsey wrote of the moment later:

"We were pretty sad, but we felt as though we were facing that painful memory of that awful day last June head on. Some people may question why we would go there. Dirk's response to that was 'Well, what if next year or the year after I am racing and I haven't been there yet. I may break down and not be able to finish the race.'"

We flew back to Honolulu for the next step—a visit to Queen's. If watching the race had been tough for me, Queen's, the site of so much devastation for Kelsey, was much worse for her. In fact, it was not tough for me at all. I didn't remember a thing about Queen's. Kelsey wanted badly to return there, to see it all again with a more lilting presence that those dark days of a year before. This time I was at her side, walking and talking, not comatose and plugged into machines keeping me alive.

I was a smiling, walking, and vibrant reminder of rare success for those critical care nurses and doctors who greeted us. More often than I'm sure they care to think about, the results of their hard work are not so visible. They do not see a great number of happy survival stories. Traumatic brain injuries do not often end with uplifting results.

Kelsey later summed up how she felt about the staff at Queen's in an earlier note to our friends, who by then included everyone on the hospital staff:

"The words 'thank you' don't seem big enough to reflect how grateful I am. The Hawaii team gave Dirk their hearts and souls—and because of that they performed a miracle. I truly believe Dirk is with us today because of the amazing care we received there."

A year later, she was able to embrace them and express those heartfelt sentiments in person—with me at her side.

Kelsey had spent a lot of wrenching, unremittingly tense times at Queen's. Our anniversary visit was a relief to her. Stepping back into that hospital room again helped her realize that she had not only survived but had overcome an enormous challenge that could have crushed her emotionally. Knowing that she had had the strength to make it through those dark weeks must have been vindicating for her—a nice acknowledgement that she was strong and collected and calm and responsive. It was a victory for her that she in fact managed very well.

A year before, doctors had asked her in that same room if I had a living will—then had told her she should be prepared if necessary to pull the plug that night.

There I was, a year later, walking the halls beside her. It was a beautiful and elating moment when we walked in the door, both for Kelsey and me and for the jubilant staff, who smothered us with hugs and kisses and shrieks of happiness.

One nurse pulled me aside and told me how glad she was to see me, and to see that I seemed to have kept my "happy prankster" personality. She recalled a night I awoke and called her to my bedside.

"I need to speak to my brother Olaf now," I had told her.

She had reminded me that it was two in the morning and that my brother might not be awake.

"Can't it wait?" she asked.

"I need Olaf—now," I said.

Olaf, who was staying in a hotel three blocks away, rushed to the hospital so fast he did not put on his shoes. He arrived panting and barefoot and I would guess alarmed that his brother needed him.

He rushed to my bedside.

"Dirk, what is it? What's wrong?"

"Can you change the channel?" I asked, pointing to the television mounted on the wall above my bed.

My love of teasing and mischief had still been there at Queen's, even though in most ways, I was not.

When we returned home after our anniversary trip, Kelsey and I both felt cleansed in some fashion. A month after our return, Kelsey was in an introspective mood when she wrote to our friends:

"Life is continuing to move forward. Last year was filled with so many heartaches, and unfortunately they just don't go away after the one-year marker. I do think, though, that time heals and we are starting to handle things a bit better. I know Dirk has a lot of anger and sadness inside him. There are days he feels everything (besides me) was taken away from him—job, athleticism, driving, independence. We tell him he has made an incredible recovery, but it's not good enough for him. He wants more and I hope that keeps him motivated. In the last few weeks he has started running on his own and one day last week he even went by himself for a bike ride on the path. He just keeps getting better. It's just very, very slow."

During the first year we had also endured another medical scare, as if the first one were not enough. A routine checkup after the tumor was removed had prompted doctors to wonder if another one was growing.

That news felt, as Kelsey put it, "like being kicked in the stomach for the second time." To me, it was as welcome as a kick about four inches farther down from my stomach. Hearing the news from the doctor was the last thing we were expecting.

I had had several MRIs over the year to watch it, vigilance always being the best way to proceed in these things. A September 2007 scan showed there had been no growth, and it appeared we were off the hook. But the whole situation was a doubled-edged sword. We were happy to get the results. Hearing you don't have a tumor is always good news. But then the waiting begins anew. Will it start growing?

Kelsey wrote of the dilemma:

"Dirk had an MRI in early September and everything looked the same—there is no growth in the area where the suspected tumor was located. This good news allows Dirk to go six months until his next follow-up appointment. I don't think waiting for the results will ever get easier. The process is stressful on both of us because you either get good news or bad news, which means our lives may potentially change in one moment."

But we had become strong, gracefully numbed to sudden blindsides of bad news:

"I don't question our ability to handle change or difficult situations, but I would rather not be faced with having to dig really deep for strength at this point. I'm still recovering from last year—as is Dirk. He is reminded daily of what he's lost, but he finds the strength every day to persevere and try new things."

We had dug deep enough, we had reinforced and strengthened our emotions and deepened our reserves. But we had enough of that. We wanted to move on.

And I had moved on, and after Hawaii I moved even further along.

By the time we were debating the trip to Hawaii, I had begun walking to the gym by myself, exerting not only my legs but my independence. It was a 20-minute trip one way. I'd work out for an hour at the gym and walk home.

As my rehab progressed over that first year, I was buoyed, supported, and cajoled by my friends. They'd check in every day, and never left me sit alone for too long. It became a comfortable, helpful rhythm. Visitors, coffee, lunch, trash talk, usually followed by a walk or maybe even a swim.

I had been swimming with Paul Lundgren once a week and had worked hard on learning not to swallow half the pool. It took me nearly a full year, but I mastered it—or rather remastered it: breathe through the nose, exhale through the mouth. Eventually I was able to start doing flip turns and had increased my daily swim to a mile. It was a painfully slow mile compared with my old times, but it was a gratifying mile nonetheless.

Over that year I had developed a mental technique for motivation—not that I was short of that. I told a therapist in one session how I tried to keep engaged during the mind-numbing and repetitive physical therapy sessions. I had an imaginary person sitting next to me who knows how to do everything, I told her. That person was the old Dirk. I would try to connect to the old Dirk, to suck up his knowledge and experiences and to then use them to reproduce the movements and the sounds and the reactions that had come so naturally and subconsciously before the stroke. In effect, it was a form of visualization that I had used in the training for races.

Over the year, I had made significant progress overcoming what Kelsey described as my life as a Weeble—as in "Weebles wobble but they don't fall down." I had been fitted with prism glasses and had Botox injections, which improved my irritating double vision. My balance had improved markedly.

I also had been gradually increasing my walking distance. For most of the year it had been just that—walking and trying to stretch the distance. The whole time I was rehabbing that first year, I pestered the doctors about when I could really put the hammer down. Needless to say, there was still concern about overexertion and what that might prompt. I was relentless, though, and finally wore them down.

I got the green light to push it more than I had been. I was anxious to test my wheels after seventeen months.

At Thanksgiving in 2006, with the whole family there, we went out behind our house for a pregorging walk along the Rails-to-Trails path behind our house. It was a spontaneous decision. I started running. Everyone looked up, a bit surprised, and, caught up in it all, started jogging alongside me, whistling and whooping. Everyone ran with me in a joyful mob.

I did not even break a sweat, but that short jaunt on the path was one of my best runs ever.

Thanksgiving had a new meaning that dinner.

That Friday, Kelsey and I braved the Black Friday mobs at a Dick's Sporting Goods in San Rafael and bought some workout clothes. I wanted to make it official. If I was going to start running again, I would do it right and look the part.

Just before Christmas, I joined a team that included Kelsey and ran a five-kilometer leg of a race.

Kelsey captured that bright moment, six months out from that day in Hawaii:

"Dirk was the last to go on our team, and he had friends and neighbors surrounding him the whole time. He did so well and it was so special for all of us to be there for the moment when Dirk crossed the finish line."

Six months had passed. They were huge. It was progress.

Kelsey wrote of that moment with great happiness:

"When I look back to where we were six months ago it blows me away to see what Dirk has accomplished. And he continues to get better every day. It's difficult for us to see the small, incremental improvement, but therapists and friends are quick to point them out. I tell Dirk that there was a time, not too long ago, that if he moved his toes or gave me a thumbs up on command, I was thrilled."

During that first year, I was working my brain, taking classes at the College of Marin, though I was not ready to get in the car and drive. That became another learning experience—and a test of expanding my patience. I took the bus and got used to the slower pace. It made for long days, but long days that kept me occupied were welcome and, in an odd way, energizing.

During that year I had also gotten off the stationary bike and did a four-mile ride on my own on the Rails-to-Trails path. The jaunt was frightening to Kelsey because of my balance issues, but exhilarating to me.

I will admit I had my down moments, when I felt that my life was nothing more than therapy sessions. I grew tired of therapy and the repetition and finding the energy to keep motivated.

I would become motivated by something else that was going on.

We learned in September 2007 we were expecting twin girls. Our lives were about to change again, in a stunningly wonderful way.

Kelsey put it rather understatedly:

"We've come a long way in one year."

Twelve

BIG CHANGES

Learning Kelsey was pregnant and then planning our next chapter was a piece of cake. We'd been talking about starting a family and had been working on it for quite a while. If we had learned anything thing since the stroke, it was patience, and we knew that patience was the key to being a good parent. We would go with the joyful flow and roll with it.

Then we learned we'd be having twins.

Thinking we were ready for the next chapter or not, the news was a bit of a shock. After that explosive news, preparing for the births and waiting for the arrival of our daughters was not unlike living within forty miles of the eight different earthquake faults near Corte Madera. You know something will happen and you think you're prepared, but deep down you're not entirely sure how you'll do.

We knew having kids would involve some amount of tension. But it was not like the involuntary, crazed tensions that were dropped on us so unexpectedly in Hawaii. This time it was a welcome tension, shared with countless others who have had a child. It was not unique. That was a quiet comfort.

And we did just fine with everything, though Kelsey's pregnancy and our waiting for the new era was not without its moments.

While the news of Kelsey's pregnancy was not unexpected, it did spark a few deep breaths and some introspection on how we would deal with it, how our lives would be further changed by this joyful new circumstance.

Priorities change after you face death head on, survive, and then have to cope with the unintended consequences and detritus that follow. After the stroke I was suddenly starting all over again just learning how to walk and talk, struggling to see straight. In an odd way, I was not too far from where our daughters would be, as if we had somehow found ourselves in the same race, at the same starting line.

At this point I still couldn't drive and was nervous about riding a bike on the road. Twins? Things you once deemed major become trivial. Things you valued fade, and you look back and wonder what caused you to ever think that way. Doing well in a race, new car, job promotion and raise, who cares? When you are given your life back and then given the chance to create two more, you become perhaps a bit more introspective, if not poetic, about values and what things mean.

I did not need a reason to dig deeper as I pushed ever so slowly through my rehab, but knowing our daughters were on the way was a good jolt of positive vibes. I wanted to work toward the time when I could run regularly, long and hard, and I wanted to work on my mind, to get back the sharpness I had had before the stroke.

During Kelsey's pregnancy, we had weekly ultrasounds to record the girls' growth, which was not unlike my own progress, slow and steady and at times not easily discernible. If you looked at the ultrasounds from one week to the next, their growth would barely register. But if you glanced at a shot of them taken in the first month and put it beside one from six months later, the growth is clearly visible—astounding, in fact. That is what was going on with me, as well. If I could have ultrasounded my own progress, those shots would have shown the same thing: slow if not immediately apparent progress.

We still have those ultrasounds, the first photos in what is now an encyclopedic volume of photos of us in every circumstance you can imagine—beaches, picnics, birthday parties, dinner celebrations, skiing. There are shots of us in California, Vermont, and Connecticut. The girls are infants, toddlers, young schoolgirls. They are growing up. The common hallmark of each of those photos of the girls and me and Kelsey is the smiles. I like that.

I had gone from needing to be lifted from bed to starting to do some wobbly attempts at hiking the rutted and steeped trials around Mount Tam. Balance was an issue. I still looked like a drunk when I walked, and I still drew attention because of that, an occasional "Jesus, it's only ten in the morning and look at that guy" kind of stares. I brushed them off, tried to not let it bother me, though it did.

The physical therapists euphemistically listed my "deficits," and the list was long. But the trick was not to look at them as a whole. *The Dirk Vlieks A to Z Catalog of Defects* was not a book I was interested in reading. I decided very early on to simply knock them off one at a time. For me, the balance issues were something I preferred to make a thing of the past.

The best, most efficient way to deal with that was to practice with my new senses, to learn how to counter the dizziness and uncertain gait that had taken over from my usual sure-footed and solid strides. Before the stroke I could glide easily over the twisted roots, jutting rocks, and crumbling trails up and down Mount Tam. And I could it do at a good pace, always able to see and sense and run and adjust without ever worrying about a twisted ankle or a nice header into a tree.

Those days were over. At first, a crack in the sidewalk could put me down. Not being quick enough to lift my foot over a slightly protruding piece of concrete was a challenge. I needed to work on that if I was to make any sort of progress.

When I returned to Mount Tam, the trails were the same, but the challenges they offered were suddenly more epic. I wasn't running anymore, I was walking. But the point was, I was out there, and that was where I needed to be. Testing, annoying, scary, frustrating, yes. But it was certainly better than a treadmill in rehab, walking slowly, going nowhere, holding onto a pair of railings that did nothing to test me. It was like a younger kid on a bike with training wheels. At some point you are going to have to take them off and give it a shot.

And, of course, Mount Tam is possibly one of the most stunning places in the country. That helped. It certainly beat staring at a wall in the rehab.

I had company on those Mount Tam trails. My mother would often make the two-hour round trip over from Livermore through what we called the "four disastrous intersections" to join me. Company always makes things move faster. Pleasant conversation is a great diversion. We'd often just head out and up the trials and start talking, not paying attention to the time or to any sort of agenda. We had some great walks, invigorating and challenging. Steep rocky trails become more of a test when you are tired. Those walks were great for the balance work I needed.

From time to time, connections to my past would suddenly appear, and that was comforting, as well —knowing my friends were along to help bridge the chasm between the old Dirk and the new. My friend Anke Teigler and her husband, Stefan, stopped in and stayed with my mother for a while and joined us on those hikes. Stefan and I had played tennis together in Germany. She worked for Interpol, and they had been living at the time in Tunisia. My support team was truly global, I guess.

I also kept my appointments moving with the Lundgrens at Presidio Sports, again focusing on the balance issue but also on strengthening my core, abdomen stuff, which we knew would help. I also expanded my weightlifting and swimming work-outs. And just in case I decided to slack off, Kelsey hired a personal trainer for me, a great guy named Pepe.

We had babies on the way, after all, and I would need as much strength and endurance as possible.

The whole time I pushed ahead, there was still a shadow. I could not turn my head quickly from one side to the other without become uncontrollably dizzy. That ruled out driving until we could find a way to clear up the problem. It also ruled out riding my bike on the street. With essentially no peripheral vison, there was no way I would be able to see a car coming up from behind me—not such a great idea with the traffic around Corte Madera.

I did take to the trails behind our house on a mountain bike Hans had given me. But even that proved precarious. I was out one afternoon, probably going faster than I should have been, when my front wheel caught a rut and I went headfirst over the handlebars. When the bike and I came down, my right calf slid across the front gear cog, making a nice, bloody gash. The funniest thing about the whole mishap was that when I went to the emergency room for stitches, I found out my tetanus immunization had expired and I needed a shot. How many hospitals had I been in by that time? How many days and weeks and procedures?

I walked everywhere, to my sessions at Presidio, to my workouts with Pepe, and to the hospital to meet with Kelsey for the ultrasounds. I developed a very pleasant morning routine. After a workout, I would walk into town, grab a nice hot cup of dark Kona coffee and a croissant, and sit at a sidewalk table and watch the world go by.

I enjoyed it immensely, though the frequent packs of cyclists heading down Palm Avenue, many of whom I knew, got under my skin. I missed that. I wanted it back.

But that became secondary as Kelsey's pregnancy progressed. Everything was secondary to getting ready for the girls. Getting my balance back, running a race well, riding the bike in traffic, doing a full triathlon—those things would come in time, I hoped. The physical therapy had become routine and predictable.

Having twins in matter of months was not.

As we prepared, other realities were becoming impossible to ignore. Our house on Palm was small, around 1,000 square feet. It was actually a modest bungalow in another time, when real estate prices in Marin County were closer to Earth. Prices were stratospheric by the time we bought it after it was expanded and renovated. With both of us working good jobs and no kids or debts to speak of, we could afford it. I loved its warmth. It was what the realtor called "comfortable." Realtors did well in Marin in those days, and in those days even "comfortable" brought in big bucks.

Kelsey continued to work at Kentfield, but as I improved and the girls' arrival approached, the Big Question that had been slumbering in the background started to become hard to ignore. Is the house too small? How will we manage twins when even the cats sometimes made things seem cramped? How will we manage to take care of two babies while I'm still rehabbing and at home? That, of course, forced the other Big Question to the surface. By then we knew progress to recovery—as steady as it was—would be slow. We knew it would be a while before I could work again.

Our prestroke days were carefree financially. It was just the two of us in a small house we could afford. We were not the tightwads of the type who folded our paper lunch bags to use again the next day, but we were not extravagant, either. We lived well but not pretentiously. But two new babies and one fewer job would present a challenge we could not ignore. Knowing I would not be working again for a while, it was becoming clearer we'd have to move.

I loved Corte Madera, but I loved a lot of things I could no longer do.

We knew, at some point, we'd be moving, and Connecticut, where Kelsey's mother and father lived with their spouses, seemed like a great place to settle. But first, we would have the twins, who as Kelsey's pregnancy developed into the noticeable stage we began calling Baby A and Baby B.

It is always tough to predict San Francisco's quirky weather, where you can sometimes experience winter and summer on the same day. But as fall slowly faded, we were ready for anything, especially the great wonder of having kids. The normal new parental anxiety faded just as fall did. Kelsey's extending abdomen made it very clear the girls were on the way. We were ready.

We had gone through the requisite prenatal course for new expectant parents, where the process is explained clinically. We knew Anna and Ellie would be delivered by cesarean, so the anxiety of breaking water and pushing and making sure to get to the hospital on time were moot. But I still listened to instructions about my role as the caring observant father who would coach his wife through the painful contractions and support her, somehow magically making the pain of childbirth disappear. The father's role in the wondrous and miraculous process of birth is to be a model of comfort and support. I'm not sure why the course designers insisted on that. I don't think it works.

It certain did not work for us.

To prepare for the births, the night before, I did what I usually did before a big race. Maybe it was superstition, maybe habit, but I had always cut my hair as short as I could. I doubt I had ever really done a good job of it, but for whatever reason, my prebirth haircut job was worse than anything I had ever done.

Kelsey had other things on her mind that day, of course, and had not noticed my new coif until we got in the car to head to the hospital. She took one look and was neither pleased nor complimentary in her comments.

We arrived at the hospital on time, parked, and announced ourselves as Kelsey's contractions began. Kelsey was ushered into the presurgery waiting room and connected to monitors that would gauge the timing and strength of the contractions to better schedule the surgery.

Now, I have always been a gearhead. I'm fascinated with computers and monitors and readouts and all that sort of stuff, and I had always used those metrics in my training. I liked being able to quantify things. I became a bit overenthusiastic about the readings marking Kelsey's contractions. Higher numbers meant more powerful contractions, which indicated increasing amounts of pain. I guess I was not listening to the birth class instructor when she reminded the expectant fathers about comfort and sympathy for the mother. I started watching the numbers rise on Kelsey's contractions and began getting caught up in the wonder if it all, as if higher number meant better.

As each readout jumped, I turned to Kelsey and congratulate her with, "That was a great one!" "Nice job!"

My enthusiasm was not well received.

Very soon after my third or fourth enthusiastic congratulation, Kelsey turned and asked me to shut up, though not as delicately as I am noting here.

A few minutes later, distracted by my inability to monitor her increasing contractions, I suggested that it was perhaps time to nail down the babies' names. That was met not with any sort of comment, but rather a look that made it very clear that any further comments from me would not be welcome.

The births went as expected, and Anna and Ellie emerged as the perfect daughters we knew they would be on February 1, 2008. All the planning and prenatal classes and advice from other parents cannot prepare you for the wonder of seeing your children for the first time. We were awed and ecstatic.

Anna and Ellie were tiny when they emerged, a not unusual situation for twins. For the first week they stayed in the hospital with Kelsey in the neonatal intensive care unit. That room was so vastly different from Queen's. There were no health concerns, no edgy worry, and no anxiety. I'd walk over to see the three of them every day, unable to stop smiling.

After they came home to Palm Avenue, things continued along the path Kelsey and I had anticipated so many months before. Life was wondrously chaotic. Kelsey returned to work, I continued with my various rehabs, we had help from friends, and our knowledge that we had to move jelled with each juggled moment.

We began to solidify the inevitable, at first emotionally, just letting the idea sink in. Talking about it and making it real. Then we began the actually planning. It was tough in some ways, easy in others. We both loved the house on Palm Avenue, but it was time to move on. We loved it even more after we were able to sell it very quickly for much more than we paid for it—a final blessing from the real estate gods of Marin County.

So we decided on eastern Connecticut and the loving embraces of Kelsey's family that awaited us. With both of her parents remarried, we had two sets of grandparents nearby. And my parents would eventually join them. With each came plenty of room, built-in babysitters, and lots of loving care. Having a lot of room was also nice, of course. There is always comfort in family, and we had plenty of comfort with Kelsey's so close.

Staying at Kelsey's mother's house in Groton, we toured the staid eastern Connecticut shoreline for our new base of operations and kept driving back to the nearby town of Mystic, an old whaling port that drew us in.

We found a new development just about to be built, the surveyors and heavy equipment out carefully clearing lots between plenty of old and gracious pine groves. We chose a lot and began plans to build a new house for our new family. It was a perfect spot, quiet and only a short walk from downtown

Mystic, Long Island Sound, and the Mystic Market, where I could resume my coffee mornings over fresh muffins. It was an appealing and inviting neighborhood. Soon enough we would learn that we would have plenty of apparently fertile neighbors with the same idea in mind—it's a perfect *Leave It to Beaver* kind of place to raise kids. Anna and Ellie would soon have dozens of friends their age to play with.

It was a good time to move on, in so many ways.

Thirteen

AN IDEA TAKES SHAPE

The move east was in no way an attempt to escape the reality of what had happened, but it did etch a distinctive line marking past, present, and future. There is no geographical cure for eluding things you would prefer to forget, but there was something about Mystic we immediately embraced—a freshness and a new energy, I guess. I had crossed the country and crossed that line.

We put the future in front of us, determined to get moving on the right course. Moving anywhere is good when you feel mired by circumstance, and there were ghosts hovering over Palm Avenue.

In Mystic, we had two beautiful and growing daughters and a great nuclear family nearby to help. I had basic goals I wanted to attend to and another more ambitious one that I had kept to myself. The basic goals, of course, centered on improving each item on the wide and varied list of damages, if not knocking them off the list, at least shrinking them. I also wanted to put behind me what was becoming the numbing reality of rehab exercises. They were beginning to seem to have no purpose, no goal.

The treadmill running, the slow jogging and slow laps in place in the pool, the sessions on the stationary bike had one thing in common: a lot of movement that went nowhere. No matter what I did, I ended up in the same place. I wanted to move ahead. I wanted a destination, some purpose for all the effort. I did not want my life to be a treadmill.

When I first started waking up at Kentfield, still not able to even get out of bed, something began flickering. It was a brief flash, there, then buried as I ever so slowly began to absorb the enormity of what had happened. In the relative scale of things, it was inconsequential at first and overcome by events that were more pressing.

It would intrude from time to time. I had never finished the race. The simple realization was really nothing more than an asterisk on a long-forgotten race list. As I improved and the larger life-and-death issues receded, it grew. And as it grew, it began to chafe. It rubbed me the wrong way and in certain moments annoyed me to no end. It was like starting a sentence and not being able to finish because someone keeps interrupting. It was unlikely anyone else actually cared about it, but I did. I detested that thing.

At Kentfield, of course, I had other things to distract me from that thought, like crawling out of bed and learning how to drink from a glass and chew and swallow my food. Later there was the surgery and all the drama that went with it. Then there were the births and the talk of moving and other more vital decisions to make. These were all worthy distractions, wonderful markers of progress.

The Did Not Finish was farther down on the list of things that rented space in my head, but it would pop up from time to time and taunt me. It was not as if I were going to have a heart-to-heart with Kelsey about it while she helped me get out of bed. She had other things on her mind, as well, like a husband who had almost died and needed constant attention as he worked his way back.

I parked the DNF, but I knew where it was. It was like the small pebble that somehow finds itself between your toes on a long run. At first you ignore it, not wanting to stop and shake it from your shoe. But after a while you have to because it's rubbing your foot raw and screaming at you.

I would finish that race.

I had been to Mystic on meet-the-family visits with Kelsey, but settling in, knowing we were not packing in three days and heading back home to California, was a new reality. Connecticut was home now. California was just a place we used to live. Connecticut was Kelsey's turf, and she knew it well. I was comfortable immediately, and Kelsey knew I would be. The old whaling port was small and bustling in its neatness, our neighborhood filled with young couples, and about to burst with kids. It was tranquil and convenient, and we felt at home immediately.

Mystic is actually and officially a village, with fewer than 5,000 people. It's in eastern Connecticut, sitting calmly on Long Island Sound, its gritty working harbor days long since replaced neatly by Mystic Seaport and its museum and nearby aquarium that attract people from across the country. We settled easily into our new house on Hatch Street, and just as easily into a welcoming routine. The Mystic Market, just down the road, around the corner on Route 1, where I could grab a cup of coffee and a muffin after a workout, reminded me of California.

We could walk anywhere we wanted, which was a welcome and planned feature of moving to Hatch. Stores, the market, groceries, anything, really, were a twenty-minute walk from home. And my all-important coffee was always within striking distance. I love my coffee and will admit under torture that I'm a bit of a snob about it.

We quickly—instantly—fell in love with the neighborhood. It was almost like every one of us had somehow all attended the same "Now it's time to settle down and have children" lecture. There was instant karma with our neighbors. The number of kids along the tree-lined and open street who were the same age as Anna and Ellie was almost freaky—but in a wonderful way. They had a ready-made gang before we had even unpacked, and as they grew older the bonds they formed were amazing to watch. Hatch is a throwback to a time long gone from our insular commuter world where neighbors don't have time to say hello. It's a place where we watch over one another and the kids and actually know our neighbors.

Kelsey quickly found a job at Lawrence + Memorial Hospital in New London, a twenty-minute drive from Mystic. We found day care for the girls. Kelsey and I had much work to do.

I was not in the clear by any means, but things were slowly improving. My vision and balance problems would insert themselves at inopportune times, and I still had to accept that the uninitiated passerby would sometime assume immediately I was drunk as I walked past them. Having that assumption from strangers became more acute at certain times, like when pushing the girls in a stroller at ten in the morning. I had grown inured to the stares, but the indignity of it all when I was with the girls was difficult to swallow.

That aside, things were starting to click, like finding that small jigsaw tile to finish a troubling corner of a complicated puzzle. There were still a lot of pieces left to find. But I was off the starting line anyway.

My affection for California notwithstanding, the Mystic move was an enthusiastic and conscious choice, obviously. We had built-in and loving day care partners with two sets of grandparents who lived just minutes way. At first, that did not include my own parents, who were still in California. Even that would change later when they, too, pulled up their California roots and moved nearby.

But even the best intentions of doting grandparents don't work every day. There were some mornings when Kelsey would have to scramble to get the kids to day care and make it to Lawrence on time. I knew I needed to get back behind the wheel, but the challenges of driving had made me procrastinate a bit. I had tried in California, and it had been an adrenaline-inducing experience, not just for me, but for my driving instructor. With my vision still blurred, I found it much easier to stay on the road—and these were busy California roads—by lining up the driver's side wheels of the car on the center line. This is not necessarily recommended or comforting for a passenger, or for anyone coming in the other direction.

On the way out to Connecticut, visiting Kelsey's brother in Cincinnati, I actually took his car for a spin one night and managed to stay mostly on the right side of the road and deal with the conventional clutch and stick shift. My coordination was fine even if my vision was still a bit suspect.

In Connecticut, the motivation to start helping in the child transportation department trumped my lack of confidence, and I realized I needed to take a shot at getting my license. Kelsey drove me to the Connecticut Department of Motor Vehicles office in Old Saybrook, where I stood in line to get a number, then sat and waited with a group of nervous high school kids and their parents. I imagine Kelsey felt the same way as those parents—nervous, proud, and resigned to the fact that there were many driving adventures ahead. I had no problem with either the written or road test, and my vision was just fine, or at least good enough to pass. Good enough to drive Anna and Ellie to day care when the need arose.

I had other things to attend to as things began to slowly knit together. One was my concentration and focus, which were shaky at times, especially when I was tired or being bombarded with too many things at once.

Kelsey's father had a friend with similar problems. A stroke victim, as well, though thirty years older, he had been taking "brain training" classes in Mystic and had told Fred that they worked very well. We signed up for classes, which were right down the road.

The euphemism-inclined medical profession called these predictable episodes of mental confusion "cognitive challenges." Why not? During a stroke, your brain has in effect spontaneously combusted and rerouted tens of thousands of finely tuned neural roadways into dead ends and misdirected pathways. Stroke victims who have reached the point where they can take "brain training" classes are the lucky ones.

I would drive myself to the Mystic Medical Center on Clara Drive twice a week and join a group of enthusiastic patients, all of whom were old enough to be my parents—a reminder that there were very few stroke survivors my age.

It was also a reminder that I had a long life ahead of me and much work to do to live it well.

Many people struggle with attention deficit disorder, with taking long and wandering mental trips along twisting backroads. "What are we having for dinner?" can send them off wondering what the gross national product of Chile is. With stroke victims, it is worse and often regular—and not so comical.

The sessions were designed to calm the mind, to teach you how to better process the sometimes jumbled thoughts and unannounced and uninvited interruptions. Exercises in the hour-and-a-half sessions would work on recognizing keys, and taking those keys and using them to focus. With help, we'd all be better able to keep on the right, clearly focused road.

These cognitive challenges can be debilitating and exhausting. Not being able to remember a simple sequence or something that happened yesterday can beat you down. Worrying about when the next time it will happen further compounds the issue. It can get out of control and become self-defeating it you let it. It was not about to.

We worked together, concentrating on how to better recognize body language, on stretching our attention spans, on problem solving, on using outside signals to focus. I had worked with computers. My mind was wired for logic and order and hierarchy of thought, for being able to make deliberate and clean transitions from one step to another. I needed to get that back, and my brain training sessions were great steps in the right direction

Naturally, as my focus began to slowly reappear, so did the DNF and my desire to make it go away.

Even as we unpacked on Hatch Street I was planning my return to Kona. I did not blare it out or make a definite pronouncement with the date and my projected finishing time.

After you've had a stroke and brain surgery, the word *definite* is not one you use with any seriousness. We had faced too many uncertainties by then to be definite about anything.

I knew I was definite about trying as hard as I could. It was all I could do. I still had a long uphill road ahead.

All the larger, more imposing obstacles aside, I also knew that announcing to Kelsey that I was heading back to Kona and the race would not be a wise way to promote marital harmony. I would wait for the right time.

I joined a master's swimming program at the Mystic Y and began taking longer runs into the hills to the north of town. Like-minded people attract one another, and I very quickly became part of the Mystic fitness community.

As I began to ease my way into this welcoming group, I did notice a change from my California days. Perhaps pushed by how close I had come to the very edge and by my need to soak in every second—with Kelsey, with the girls, with life itself—I slowed down.

In the ancient history of my training—the Before the Incident Days—I would push it every single day. I had never cared how I would finish a race as long as I knew I had pushed as hard as I could. When I trained I made sure I could do that. Training runs or swims or bike rides were always to the max. That was the only way I knew how.

When I settled back into it in Mystic, the high voltage was gone. My goal of finishing Kona was there and becoming more pronounced, but how I would get to the starting line, how I would prepare, had become less electrified. I'd train for it, and train hard, but if I felt like taking a day off, I would. If I felt like easing up on the final hundred yards in a swim workout, I would. I had been incapable of doing that in California.

It was never a conscious decision. I didn't wake up one morning and say, "I'm not putting the hammer down any more." It just slowly overtook me. When I started training again, my goals were different—I was different. I wanted to finish the race, period. I did not want to beat my old times or do better splits or a faster swim. I wanted only to cross the finish line.

There was still much to do with balance and speech issues and many other things, but I now had a focus.

I would point to that focus but I would take deep breaths, inhaling every single thing during every single day. I did not need brain training to reach that epiphany.

Fourteen

THE RETURN

For me, June 4, 2011, was another day at the office. I was a journeyman Lazarus, rising slowly from the explosion and the destruction it had caused. I was there to finish what I had started, to complete the circle.

I had been bolstered by hard work and the fragile, often fleeting hopes of others. I was heading for the starting line to erase a moment suspended in heartbreak that had hung over so many people I loved for five years. That was far too long for that sort of pain. I wanted to begin a fresh and vibrant new chapter of my life.

We would all see how it turned out.

The day began with promise. By sunset, the results would likely mean different things to the many people who had been with me along the way. They would all have one thing in common as the day began. They were all taking short nervous breaths, waiting to exhale a soothing gust of relief if things turned out well.

This day, I knew, was for my father, who had called learning of my collapse "the worst day of my life." It was for Kelsey, who had been told to be prepared to end my life and who had been with me every second since. It was for Jimmy Riccitello, who had found me on the side of the road, and the doctors in the medical tent and the staff at Queen's. The day would lie tensely in front of Hans and everyone at Kentfield and the many friends on the long list of email supporters who egged me on and offered prayers and hope.

As I walked down to the beach in Hawaii, I knew that what I was trying to do that day would drop many of my loved ones into a state of hopeful tension. There would be prayers, no doubt, to please, please not let it happen again. *Please don't put us through the chaos and pain again.*

The stroke had shocked so many people dear to me, had sparked many tears and pit-of-the-stomach terrors. It had, I knew, prompted two-in-the-morning moments of despair, of paralyzing sadness and farewells to dreams that would not be fulfilled. It had been ugly. But it was real. It had happened, and nothing could be done to make it disappear. All I could now was work to smooth the rough edges torn from the middle of my life. I was fine with that. Look back at the past, just don't stare. Don't live in it, because it is not coming back.

I wanted the camera in my imaginary movie to focus on the moment in the medical tent when Kelsey had noticed my bare legs splayed on the table, my mouth agape—the instant our lives changed forever. I wanted that scene to be cut and edited out. I wanted it replaced with a new scene, where I emerged from the tent, smiled, dusted the Queen K dirt from my jersey, got back on the bike, and finished the race.

That is why I was walking down the beach to the start.

Five years sounded right, not because a cosmic numerological voice spoke to me, but because things just worked out that way. I had worked toward it, and I felt I was ready. I am not a big believer in numerology. I had not geared myself at Kentfield for a Hollywood-moment return on the fifth anniversary. I am not a big believer in Hollywood moments. It just happened. Make no mistake, it was glorious to walk down the beach for the start of the swim, and I sucked in every sparkle of it. I was calm, but very motivated to put this thing to rest.

Jimmy Riccitello was there. So was race director Diana Bertsch. So were Kelsey and my parents and Charlie Ehm. There were others who were there five years earlier, when instead of crossing the finish line I was prone in the medical tent, so very close to the edge. Five years later, all across the country, my friends were wondering how I'd do as they went about their distracted workdays, waiting for a text or an email saying that I had done it, that I had finished and was still alive—that I had not pushed it too far.

I am certain my supporters at the race that day were all more nervous than I was. And they would stay that way, too, all day long, waiting through the various phases, breaths catching when I did not appear from the water or down the road when I should have. For my loved ones and friends, the day would be filled with darker memories forcing themselves back to the surface. A finish would close the circle. I knew they would have to be patient while I went about my work. If I crossed the finish line, they could purge every dark moment of the last five years. It would be an effervescent cleansing of so many unspoken fears.

As for me, I was just wired into making my way comfortably through each phase. I was a different triathlete by then, with far different goals and a concept of racing that would have been alien to me before the stroke. I had returned to the Honu Half in 2011 to put the annoying DNF in the hamper and slam the lid shut and lock it. I had reinforced my punch-in punch-out rules: finish the job I had started. Closing out that chapter was simply something I had to do. It was an annoying burr that had to disappear. I did not need that DNF on my shoulder, mocking me.

I still had a fairly long list of other things to check off, and I would work on them when the time came. But first, I had to finish.

As we settled into our comfortable Mystic routine, I knew I would return to Honu, but I decided I would tell Kelsey my decision later. She had been through too much, her emotions were still tender and fragile and often very close to the surface when she spoke of those days. The stroke had been more devastating to her than to me. She lived through every second of it while I remembered nothing of the race or of Queen's. It was difficult for her to even think about it, let alone speak of it. But of course she had to, far too many times. People were sometimes mildly curious about her husband, sometimes abrasively rude. Kelsey was the one who had to deal with it.

Until I could show her I was fit enough to try, telling her I was going back to Honu and the race would have been thoughtless, possibly even cruel. I still had work to do to get to that point.

Kelsey and I both had work to do, and Anna and Ellie had school and new friends and many new things to jump into.

We were no different from any other family on Hatch Street. My job was to get better, to improve physically and sharpen my mind, and I accepted the assignment as I did every other job I had ever had. I would do the best I could.

By then, the girls were growing old enough to take in the world around them, to wonder about things in only the way young minds can wonder. I wanted to make sure they never wondered about their father. I was not going to be the sullen guy who sat moping in his chair and never went anywhere. I refused to be angry. Anna and Ellie would see only a joyful, positive father who laughed with them and filled their lives with happiness. And it would not be an act.

I could have gone down that path. I imagine many people, friends and strangers, might have even accepted that. Dirk has had a tough break, no wonder he's strung so tightly. The girls would not have understood that. They would never see anything vaguely resembling self-pity from me.

So I went to work seriously. The master's swimming program at the Mystic Y was just as important to me as my first day on the job at iBeam Broadcasting. Effort will always produce rewards, and there was no reward I wanted more than sending that DNF into oblivion.

I was still unable to do even a single a lap without drinking half the pool. My balance and thus my road biking was still suspect. I got a stationary trainer I could lock my bike into and I'd ride in the garage, the door open on nice days, looking out onto Hatch Street. By then I could ride hard for hours, but only with the security and steadiness provided by the trainer's stability. Riding out on the road in traffic was an adventure I was not ready for when we first moved in.

Running, on the other hand, was fine. In Mystic I began to hit my stride. When I ran, the slight stumbling hitch that had worked its way into my walk disappeared. Running, I looked like my old self. My running appeared close to fluid. If I had run through town instead of walking, I would never have gotten those judgmental stares, the "what's wrong with him?" looks that would be occasionally thrown my way.

I began training the way I wanted to train—for a reason, with a goal. I knew where I was planning to go, but I said nothing to my fellow swimmers or the growing group of friends I would run with all over town and beyond. It was a great group, and we immediately fell into the comfortable rhythms of talking trash and the subtle pushiness that runners who know one another well use as motivation. We jived with great enthusiasm and little sympathy, but I was not about to tell them I was going back to Honu.

The group in Mystic was like any group I had ever joined in anywhere else I had lived. I fit in right away, as I knew I would. As soon as you tie your shoes and hit the road in anything that looks like a regular pattern, you will begin to see the others doing the same thing. It did not take me long to fall in with the group of hard-core runners in Mystic.

Jim Roy, John Fox, and Dave Menze wasted very little time before they started to push me, to goad me in the way that competitive runners who like one another and enjoy one another's company do. There is not a lot of subtlety to it. These guys were no different from my friends in California, and I suspect there is some sort of law of universal attraction when it comes to runners everywhere. We run, therefore we like one another, therefore we give one another as much verbal abuse as we can.

John Fox was crazy competitive. He is the type of guy who thinks he's had a bad run if he wasn't fighting off nausea at the end. He was always happy if he bent over and gave up his breakfast after a run. He seemed to think that meant he had done enough. It was an instinct he could do nothing to control, and he knew it.

John was fast, too. John lived on Montauk Road in Mystic, a long, gradual slope that if approached on the downhill pretty much yelled out to runners to go all out. Like me, John was a numbers and gadget guy. There was nothing he would not strap on or wire himself into that he wouldn't try. I'm the same way. I love monitoring devices and the hard data they offer. You can't say, "I had a good run today" when your wrist monitor points out you did not.

We soon began using Strava software to compete, even when we were not running with each other. The downhill mile in front of his house was the perfect stretch. And the thing about Strava is it not only gives you an exact time for a certain stretch, if you program it, it will send an email message with your results to anyone you choose. We chose each other, and soon enough the electronic trashing began.

Dirk Vlieks has taken your crown.

"Hey John, I see you weren't feeling well today. I hope everything is OK."

John was good motivation, and a good prod for what I had in mind.

The master's class was the same. Swimming with a formal group provides a motivation you simply cannot produce on your own, no matter how much you try or how much you convince yourself that you're pushing it hard. With a group you have to keep up, you have to match certain times and do a fixed amount of laps in a fixed amount of time. And you get the added benefit of coaching and advice on improving technique. I was still swallowing more water than I should have been, but the push of the group and the sheer repetition of swimming had cut it back.

My confidence grew, though I was still swimming in a pool. So was my still unspoken goal of returning to Hawaii.

I knew at some point I would have to get outside and swim in the more chaotic laboratory of a lake or the ocean. The start of any triathlon, the swim, if viewed from a distance looks very similar to a feeding frenzy of piranha right after someone throws a bloody side of beef into a placid lake. Swimming at the start of a large triathlon feels like you are the middle of it, too. I needed to test myself for that one.

My plan was to first introduce the idea of my doing a triathlon by signing up for a sprint in nearby Niantic. It would get me back in the swing of things, and it would plant the seed for Honu. Niantic's short course—half-mile swim; twelve-mile bike; three-and-a-half-mile run—was a perfect distance for my return to racing.

The biggest challenge even for Niantic was the bike—not the distance, but simply keeping my balance and not drifting across the road or off it into a tree. Kelsey unwittingly helped me with that one.

One of the contractors helping finish the house, Nick, happened to be a top-notch cyclist. She asked him to lead me on the bike leg of the race, providing a target to follow. He can ride in front of you and keep you in line, she said to both of us one afternoon. Nick is a Cat 2, just short of professional, which means he can crank it out. In Niantic, he started out slowly. I'm sure he's thinking, *The guy has had a stroke, I need to take it easy.* I quickly disabused him of that notion though, riding behind and yelling at him to pick up the pace.

All the laps in the pool, the hilly running, the hours on the bike in the garage came with something I had not been seeking. My entire outlook had changed. I was back in the stream again, but this time my goal was not to beat anything: my old time, the guy in front of me, or whatever else I had used before to get motivated. My goal this time was simply to finish. Finishing was good. I had come so close to not finishing anything. I had many things I wanted to finish, and racing was just one. Like life itself, I wanted to finish with grace.

Having everything in my life I had so carefully planned derailed so suddenly and completely had given me the gift of knowing there was no need to hurry. Positive things will happen if you don't panic, set goals, and work. I wanted to put the DNF behind me and move on. I had many things I wanted to put behind me. Honu was just the tip of the list.

My entire philosophy had changed. Nearly dying has a way of altering plans. In California, I would feel guilty if I skipped a workout, and as a result I rarely did. In Connecticut, if I looked out the window and saw it was sleeting or sloppy, I was more inclined to skip heading out. I was fine with taking a day off from time to time, with slowing down and taking a deep calming breath—to relish the simple joy of being alive. That was all very good to me. I had been blessed despite the darkness.

After I crossed the line in Niantic on August 8, 2010, I knew I was ready, and I knew I had to break the news to Kelsey. I would return to Kona, and I would try to close out the unfinished business that had gnawed at me for five years. When I finally told her, she knew immediately that this was not "I might return to Kona" or a "maybe I'll return to Kona." She knew I meant it and realized I had been planning it all along. She was not surprised and understood that when I said I would do something, I would follow through.

The next Honu was less than a year away.

I knew I would do everything possible to finish, and I hoped I would. There was a difference, though. When I next stood on the beach at Hapuna, I would not be at the front of the throng of swimmers. I'd be at the rear, contented. I would not be champing at the bit up front, ready to take the inevitable elbows and kicks to the face. I'd be with the gentler folks in the rear—the ones without the anxiety and the nerves.

Before we left Mystic for the flight out, the *New London Day* ran a feature on my plans to finish the race that had nearly killed me.

By then Kelsey was fine with the idea, and philosophical about where we were before heading back to Hawaii.

"Kelsey and Dirk said they are both looking forward to getting back to the race despite what happened there in 2006," the reporter wrote.

"Hawaii has been a special place for us," Kelsey said. "It could have been much worse. It could have happened to him in the water or during those hundreds of miles on the bike in the weeks before the race. He was looked after that day.

"So we need to say 'thank you' to this place."

Kelsey added that she wasn't worried about me.

"I totally trust Dirk. I've been hard on him to get out there on the bike. He's done the swimming and the running. He's strong enough to get through this," she said. "And everyone working on the race will be looking out for him that day.

"It's going to be emotional. But I'll put on a good smile most of the time."

On June 4, 2011, I was on the beach at the back, as planned. Kelsey and the rest of my family waited anxiously, the past five years pressing heavily down. Emotions were taut, but no one said a thing, just offering wan smiles and nervous encouragement. I suppose they were all silently pushing back the memories that were trying to force their way to the surface. But they were all prepared and hoping for the best.

Some might have been thinking about the bike ride I took with Diana Bertsch the day before. Diana was not encouraged by the drifting line I took and my occasional wobbling. She had not seen me ride since that day five years before and was worried. In fact, she had mentioned to a few friends that it seemed like a bad idea for me to do the race, that it might be too dangerous. But in her role as race director she did nothing. She knew how much I wanted this.

The morning of the race was nothing short of beautiful. It was sunny, with just a whisper of an offshore breeze and a thin wreath of clouds on the horizon. There was a faint mist that promised good weather and flat water for the swim. That was a welcome sight, since a choppy surface would have been challenging with my swallowing problems.

As the crowd gathered on Hapuna Beach for the swim start, I had my body marked and stowed my eyeglasses on a nearby table. A few days before as I stared from the beach, the water had seemed big and uninviting. On race day it was welcoming. I worked my way to the back, as I had planned. I was calm and determined but must admit I was absorbing the vibe and feeling the excitement. It had been a while, and I had missed it more than I realized.

I took a quick dip to get my pulse up, then worked my way once again to the back. I took in the nervous crowd of swimmers surrounding me and felt good.

The planets were aligned.

After the usual thrashing at the start, even toward the back with the supposedly gentler people, my nerves settled about a quarter mile in. I fell into a rhythm I would keep for the rest of the day.

I felt very good, even though I had done maybe half the training I would normally have done. That was a gift, as well, being relieved of that constant pressure to do more things faster.

I was out of the water and putting on my glasses for the bike ride in just over fifty minutes, and I was fine with that, especially since I had not swallowed half the bay. My last Honu, where I had been driven to qualify, I had finished the swim in a half hour. I was not concerned. I wanted only to pace myself, and I knew how to do that. I would not push, and I would finish.

In fact, on the bike ride, I did something I would never have considered in the past. It would have been unadulterated sacrilege. Ten minutes in, I pulled over and stopped at a roadside porta potty for a break. I needed to go, so I did.

The bike leg was an out-and-back. I had not given it too much thought, but somewhere along the line I did wonder how it would feel to pass the spot where I had crumbled five years before. It would have been poetic to have literally put it behind me. But the "spot" was no longer part of the course. The turn-around point had been moved back. I caught a quick glimpse of it out of the corner of my eye and thought very briefly about how far I had come.

I felt confident. I was not going to relive that moment again. It was over and done with. I turned and rode on.

My supporters tried to keep up with my progress, tension and emotions in check though slowly percolating toward the surface. Each mile I passed brought more relief. Kelsey and Jimmy Riccitello broke form, though, the faux stoicism cracking as the long day progressed. With me on the bike, out of sight, it all became too much for them. It was, after all, on the bike that the old Dirk had vanished. Jimmy grabbed Kesley, and they took to the road on his scooter to find me and assure themselves I was still moving.

I was.

I kept a steady pace and finished the bike leg in just under four hours, almost twice as long as my usual bike leg. It was not a problem.

The run to me was easy, and I found my stride quickly, falling into a steady pace. I began to pass a few runners. The tensions of the day for my supporters were relieved briefly with a bit of comic relief. For my parents and Kelsey and anyone else looking for me, I was easy to spot. During my porta potty interlude, I had tucked some toilet paper into the back of my shorts, in case of an emergency. The tight little tissue roll I had so unglamorously stuffed in came undone and trailed me like the tail of a kite for the rest of the run.

I heard a slow and growing wave of applause wash over the people as I approached the finish line more than six hours later. As I worked my way to the tape, spectators stepped onto the course to offer high fives. It was against the rules, certainly, to step onto the course and to interact with the runners. No one cared. I had broken a lot of rules by then. The rule that you don't live after a massive stroke, the rule that you live quietly and accept your fate, the one that says you must suffocate your hopes and never, under any circumstances, in any shape or form, finish the thing that came so close to killing you.

I returned those high fives with enthusiasm, and for the first time since I had checked into work, I smiled.

I gave a quick fist pump.

I had done it. I had buried the monkey, banished it forever.

Kelsey met me at the line with a gentle hug and followed me through the finish line minglers as they reached out to offer their congratulations. As I bent over to accept my finisher's lei, she stood beside me. She had been beside me for five difficult years. There was no need for us to say a thing.

My parents, along with Jimmy Riccitello and Charlie Ehm, stood back in numb relief, smiling. It had been quite a day.

The word that I finished spread quickly within the circle of the many people who had embraced me, texts and emails flying. Dirk finished. There was likely a collective sigh of relief and no doubt a few tears. But this time they were tears of joy.

Things had worked out the way they were supposed to. That can happen sometimes.

When we returned home, *The Day* did a short follow-up piece, noting that I had finished.

"Despite still having vision and balance problems, Vlieks completed the 1.2-mile swim, 56-mile bike ride and 13.1 mile run in 1,071th place among the 1,600 competitors."

It was after that I had the first inkling that maybe I had found something to do that would transform my experience, turn it into something meaningful.

One reader responded with a note:

"Mr. Vlieks, you are an inspiration not to just those that have to overcome illness, but to all of us that have to overcome adversity. Congratulations on such a remarkable achievement. I hope your story is able to reach all those that may benefit from it."

Another added:

"You are a true inspiration to all who have had difficulties in their lives."

Inspiration sounded like a pretty good idea to me.

Fifteen

THE PATHS AHEAD

With the Honu Half and its elating, draining, and illuminating experience behind me, I took a deep breath. I had wanted to finish and I did. I had wanted my loved ones and friends to see me cross the finish line and they did. I wanted them to stop worrying about me, to see that I was fine and that I would persevere and flourish.

It was not as if I planned to retire after the finish. I could have. I could have pulled on the T-shirt, dropped the finisher's medal around my neck, and soaked up the adulation. I doubt anyone would have said a thing.

I wanted to move on. As fulfilling as it was, that finish was nothing more than a race well done. I had other races in front of me. I had closed a chapter. I had other things on my mind as I sat after the race in the warming Hawaiian sun that afternoon in Honu.

I had known even if others had not that I would finish the Honu Half upright and well. Even while I was training for it, I had started thinking of what I would do next to challenge myself physically. A marathon sounded about right. The iconic New York City Marathon was very close to Mystic. If I ran and finished a marathon, I might continue to elicit the local support I seemed to have inspired. That would blend perfectly with something else I had on my mind: to somehow use my struggle to help others.

People who knew me were aware by then that I was fine and back in working order. I had laid to rest their fears that I would somehow crumble if I exerted myself too much. They knew I had been though the blast furnace and had emerged fully formed on the other side, still strong and still resilient. I wanted to show others who might be struggling that anything is possible.

I had a few things to overcome, but to me they were minor irritations, nothing but trifling bumps in the road. Occasionally, strangers would stare as I walked, wondering if I had been drinking. It happened at a liquor store when I stopped in one morning to buy a bottle of wine for a gourmet dinner I planned to cook for my parents. It happened in Hawaii when I was helping with the Ironman. My friend Michael Carson was appalled. I told Michael and other friends who took offense to calm down. What other people thought was not my problem.

The slight shamble when I walked and my slow way of speaking as I work on enunciating clearly continue to fade, and

I continue to work on them, even today. Before Honu I had been videotaped by a local news station talking about the stroke and why I was returning to Hawaii and what I had hoped to do. I can barely understand myself in that piece, five years ago. I'm much better now and will keep getting better. That is called progress—and progress is the only thing that matters to me.

After Honu I bore down on New York, looking at life ahead as two forks in a road taking different paths. One path would be my fitness challenges, the things that had driven me before the stroke. The second path would be what I would do with the rest of what others might call "real life."

Kelsey and I had both focused on finishing a marathon in 2013, mine in New York while she wanted to run in Portland, Maine. She followed through and finished well enough to qualify the next year for Boston. I ended up pulling a hamstring and deferring New York until 2014.

The summer of 2014 was a brutal one in Mystic. It was unrelentingly hot and humid and very atypically New England. The heat never let up, and even running by the beach, hoping for a cooling breeze off Long Island Sound, brought no relief. I was determined to be ready for the November race, though, and still put in the requisite seventeen- or eighteen-mile runs at the end. I had certainly logged the miles.

Anyone who runs even occasionally will often feel they are alone, putting in the miles like no one else. These thoughts come naturally to runners spending hours on the road with nothing to do but think. As you plod along, you tend to elevate yourself as a singular athlete in a heroic pursuit of fitness. It's a motivator.

That whole image will be quickly disabused if you ever make it to the start of a New York City Marathon. On November 2, 2014, there were more than 50,000 men and women lined up in front of the Verrazano-Narrows Bridge for the start. It was one huge mass of humanity, each of whom had logged enough miles to think they were ready to race 26.2 miles more into Central Park. It was amazing and humbling.

The day before, I had taken the two-and-a-half-hour train ride into New York for the race, making the short walk over to Kelsey's father's apartment on the East side, where I spent the night. The next morning, I hopped the subway downtown and caught the Staten Island ferry over to the start. It was wondrously chaotic, seeing that mass of people getting ready to run. I was just a small dot in a huge sea, and I had managed a bit of my own chaos. In my rush to get to the start, I forgot my bib. Bibs are numbered based on how fast a runner estimates his time. Leaders, of course, go out in front of the pack, followed by progressively slower groups. By forgetting my bib, I was given a replacement that put me in the rear, with the slowest group.

Any thoughts I might have had about catching up with my own 3:30 runners quickly disappeared. It was impossible to break free.

As we headed onto the nearly-mile-long arching bridge, the entire group was hit by phenomenal 40 mph crosswinds. They were strong enough to get me thinking about being blown right into the icy waters of the Narrows separating Brooklyn and Staten Island. As a result, even with the protection of the mob surrounding me, we all headed ono the bridge at 45-degree angles to be able to move ahead.

It was an amazing and electrifying day, and my first-ever chicken-walk start to a race. It was certainly my most crowed race ever. I never broke from the group. I was like a small stick in a rapidly moving stream. There was no way to get out. I was carried along by the runners surrounding me, unable to break out or slow down.

Kelsey and my parents had agreed to meet me at Mile 17, just as the race entered Manhattan, where they had planned to cheer me on as I headed down to the finish in Central Park. Our rendezvous never happened. Just as I was approaching the spot, a woman in front of me stopped abruptly, dead in her tracks. There was nothing gradual about it. She did not slow down or even stumble. She just hit the brakes. I had no choice but to run right into her, and I nearly ran right up her back. I stumbled but managed to pull myself up by grabbing someone's bib in front of me.

Kelsey and my parents didn't even see me in the pileup. So much for my cheering section. But there was plenty of cheering, believe me. The finish at the New York City Marathon is almost an anticlimax after running twenty-six miles through all five boroughs with an uninterrupted and raucous cheering section the entre time. It seems like the entire city stops to come out and watch and urge the runners on. There is nothing like it.

As I crossed the finish line, spent but happy, I quickly realized that the relief tents where runners could get help and warm clothes and much-needed infusions of nutrition was a two-mile walk ahead. As I made my way to the tents, I passed runners who were crashing to the roadway, bonking. They had held it all together for the race but had no more to give. People were staggering as they tried to make it to the tents.

I felt fine, though I was so hungry I thought about ripping some bark off one of the trees and eating it. I had knocked off another milestone. New York was in the bag. I would do other races—maybe even Boston if I could qualify. That would put the icing on the cake.

I had other things on my mind. I had still to clear the way ahead on the other path in front of me, my real-life path.

I needed something more to do than races. Trying to qualify for Boston could wait a bit.

I had invested heavily in my recovery. I still had a way to go, and I will always have a way to go, I guess. I wanted to start getting a yield from all the work, a return on that investment that might help others facing challenges. I did not want to waste those years of recovery and be tied to small headlines in local newspapers about DIRK VIIEKS FINISHES ANOTHER RACE.

I knew I had something to offer, and I knew there had to be more than running races. I wanted to make a difference. The effort and the tears and the tensions—not just mine, but those of my friends and loved ones—had to produce something more than a few headlines about races.

I had been moved by comments from people after I had returned to Mystic from Honu. People would stop me on the street or at the market and tell me I had been an inspiration. They would talk about an uncle or a brother or a child who I had somehow perked up after hearing what I had done. I realized there were others suffering from challenges that needed a flash of hope, people who had been beaten down and needed some light. I could do that, I thought. I had plenty of light to share.

Not long after I returned from New York, I nabbed a job as assistant tennis coach at Connecticut College in nearby New London. I loved it. There was a wonderful sort of congruity to it. It made sense somehow. I think I made a difference, too. The former head case tennis player now showing his new charges that the challenges of a tennis match were minor compared with other things. Plus, I got the chance to run them into the ground with working on their fitness. I enjoyed that, and in the end they were happy about that, as well.

One of my players told a reporter from the *Norwich Bulletin*, "Our fitness has improved dramatically. He always has a new workout that he likes to torture us with; he keeps us in line that way. He's a huge inspiration. He's definitely one of the most influential people I've met at Conn. The fact that when he does take us out for runs, he's miles ahead of us."

No kidding.

But there is something else awaiting me, too, something else I could do where I would make a difference. I got a call from the principal of a local elementary school.

"I've been reading about you and have seen you running around town," he said. How would you like to give a talk to my kids? I think they'd love it."

"Sure," I said, automatically.

After I hung up, it dawned on me. I had never given a talk to kids before and did not know what to expect. I knew kids were a wild card. If I didn't keep their attention, I knew I'd be rambling on in front of a very hostile audience. Kids don't have much of a tolerance for boredom. I started to worry that it would be a fairly brutal morning if I couldn't pull it off.

Besides, what would they think about the slow and careful way I talked? They'd pick up on that very quickly. What about the way I would have to shuffle onto the stage? College tennis players and adult triathletes were one thing; bored kids were quite another.

I was more nervous driving over to the school than I had been before any race.

As I walked up to the stage, I was mortified at what seemed to be a very large group of kids. Were there really that many kids in one small school? They chatted among themselves, but as the principal called their attention to me, it became very quiet.

I eased into the talk with a video of the start of the Ironman and all its frenzy. As it ended, the kids began once again to chatter. I wasn't sure if it was the video or boredom.

"I've been in that crazy swim," I told them.

That caught their attention, and the room settled. Seeing so many swimmers kicking and fighting to get into the water had caught their attention. After that, the video over, it was showtime. I had to hold that attention.

"I've done this race," I told them. "I've been right in the middle of that mess. I've been kicked and elbowed and swallowed a lot of the Pacific Ocean."

I pulled them in a bit more, describing the race in Mystic terms. The swim was the same distance as from the drawbridge in the center of town down Route 1 to Old Mystic. The bike ride was the same as pedaling into New York City, except hillier. The run was the same as driving halfway to Providence.

"And the challenge of a triathlon is that we do these three things one after the other, as fast as we can."

I had been wrong to worry about their disinterest. They sat silently but were paying attention.

There I was, on their very own stage, a guy from town who had actually done that race. As I started talking, I told them right away that they certainly must have heard that I spoke differently. I mentioned that they must have noticed I walked with a bit of a hitch across the stage before I started.

They didn't care.

To them I was just a guy from town who had faced some sort of challenge but who had actually done this amazing Ironman thing. They saw only a guy who had the discipline and energy to train for this long and painful race. And he did it all in one day.

They did not care about the way I talked or walked.

Then I got down to what I truly wanted to share with them.

I put it in a context they would understand, so it was not about racing or even winning, or even about this guy from Mystic who had done this very cool thing. I told them about my stroke and what it had done to me. I talked about how I had to learn everything all over again, like a newborn baby. I spoke about my long recovery. Kids have no filter, they lack the guile to gloss over things the way an adult might. I put it to them directly.

"You hear the way I speak and you can see that I am different, but none of that matters. I enjoy every single day," I said. "That's my secret."

"I like challenges. Everyone has them. Some might be harder than others, but in the end, how you deal with challenges is all the same. How do you face things that might seem difficult or scare you?

"My secret is I never let anyone tell me I can't do something. I never let bullies get to me or bother me. I ignore them. Bullies hate being ignored. I hear things when people make fun of me and I don't care and don't let it bother me.

"If you are confident about yourselves, if you believe in yourselves, you will never be bullied. Confident people scare bullies."

The kids began to settle. They seemed to be listening.

"I look ahead," I said. "I absolutely never listen to people who misunderstand what I am and what I am doing. I think of what I can do, not what I cannot do.

"I don't let people and their ignorance ever get me down," I told them.

"My secret is I know I can do anything I want to if I keep trying. And that can be your secret, too. Life is about the journey and how you make it. It isn't about winning or losing, because you are going to see plenty of both. If you put your minds to it, there is nothing you cannot do."

By then the entire gym of chattering kids had grown silent.

"Get outside and try to see things you never see. Enjoy every day. Work hard. Don't judge others and try to help. It's a pretty simple secret formula," I told them.

"And now it is yours."

Then I asked if there were any questions.

Hands shot up. I had pulled them in. They had actually listened. I took questions from the kids for fifteen minutes. *What did it feel like? I've seen you running, are you going to do it again? Did it hurt? How did you learn about Ironman? Do you know the winners?*

I had hit all the right notes.

After the principal stepped out on stage and ended the flurry of questions, I walked into what seemed like a sea of enthusiasm. Kids surrounded me, wanting to talk some more, to tell me of their own runs and adventures and races.

As I headed to the door, a boy reached out and grabbed my shirt.

"You are a hero," he said, as he looked up at me.

I had not thought of it that way, but it sounded pretty good to me.

Acknowledgments

I would like to thank my co-author and friend, Tom McCarthy, for his amazing ability to help capture my story and work tirelessly with me over lots of coffee.

To our family, who all relived the events and spent hours reading drafts. They believed in the mission of portraying the accurate information to our readers. Their dedication and input to this book was necessary and very much appreciated.

To our dear friends who helped Kelsey through the darkest hours in my life and probably hers, too.

Deep thanks also to Kentfield Hospital, Presidio Sports Medicine, and Aperture Technologies for help beyond what they had to do.